Seven Steps to Reduce Fibromyalgia Therapy and Meditation: Reduce Pain, Decrease Inflammation, and Improve Sleep Quality.

By Author: Sherri Todd

Copyright @2024 by Sherri Todd

All rights reserved. No part of this publication may be reproduced, stored, or transmitted in any form or by any means electronic, mechanical, photocopying, recording, scanning, or otherwise without written permission from the publisher. It is illegal to copy this book, post it to a website, or distribute it by any other means without permission.

Sherri Todd asserts the moral right to be identified as the author of this work.

Sherri Todd is not responsible for the persistence or accuracy of URLs for external third-party internet Websites referred to in this publication and does not guarantee that any content on such websites is or will remain accurate or appropriate.

Designations used by companies to distinguish their products are often claimed as trademarks. All brand names used in this book and on its cover are trademark names, service marks, trademarks, and registered trademarks of their respective owners. The publisher and the book are not associated with any product or vendor mentioned in this book. None of the companies referenced within the book have endorsed the book.

Violators of the copyright will face the full extent of the law.

First Edition

TABLE OF CONTENTS

Seven Steps to Reduce Fibromyalgia Pain through CBT Therapy and Meditation: Reduce Pain, Decrease Inflammation, and Improve Sleep Quality 1

Introduction 7

    Fibromyalgia in Women Seniors: A Detailed Overview 9

        Epidemiology and Prevalence 9

        Understanding the Condition 9

        The Role of Hormones 9

        Unique Challenges 10

        Interactive Element: Reflecting on Your Experience 10

    1.2 Debunking Myths: What Fibromyalgia Is and Is not 11

    1.3 The Invisible Battle: Understanding the Emotional Toll 12

    1.4 Fibromyalgia and Aging: Navigating the Double Challenge 14

    1.5 Recognizing Fibromyalgia Symptoms Unique to Senior Women 16

    1.6 The Importance of Early Detection and Management 17

Chapter 2 Holistic Approaches to Managing Fibromyalgia 19

    2.1 The Role of Diet in Managing Fibromyalgia Pain 19

        Nutritional Impact on Symptoms 19

        Dietary Changes for Relief 20

        The Importance of Hydration 20

        Personalized Nutrition Plans 20

        Textual Element: Your Personalized Fibromyalgia Diet Plan 20

    2.2 Introduction to CBT: A Powerful Tool for Pain Management 21

        Basics of Cognitive Behavioral Therapy 21

        CBT for Fibromyalgia 21

        Mind-Body Connection 22

        Finding a CBT Practitioner 22

    2.3 Meditation for Fibromyalgia: More Than Just Relaxation 23

Introduction to Meditation 23

Benefits for Fibromyalgia 23

Starting a Meditation Practice 23

Resources for Guided Meditation 24

2.4 Combining CBT and Meditation: A Synergistic Approach 24

Case Studies and Success Stories 25

Developing a Personalized Plan 25

Overcoming Obstacles 25

2.5 Tailoring Your Pain Management Plan: Tips and Tricks 26

2.6 Understanding and Overcoming Common Treatment Barriers 27

Chapter 3 Cognitive Behavioral Therapy (CBT) for Fibromyalgia Pain 29

3.1 CBT Explained: Changing Pain Through Mindset 29

Understanding Cognitive Distortions 29

The Power of Thought Restructuring 29

CBT Techniques for Pain Management 29

Building a CBT Toolkit 30

Textual Element: Your Personal CBT Toolkit for Fibromyalgia 30

3.2 Identifying and Challenging Fibromyalgia-Related Negative Thoughts 30

3.3 Setting Realistic Goals and Celebrating Progress 32

3.4 Coping Strategies for Fibromyalgia Flare-Ups 33

3.5 Enhancing Self-Efficacy in Managing Chronic Pain 34

Building Confidence in Managing Fibromyalgia 35

Role of Education and Skills Training 35

Creating a Support System 35

Self-Care Practices 35

3.6 Building Resilience Against Fibromyalgia Through CBT 36

Chapter 4 Meditation Techniques for Pain Reduction 38

4.1 Getting Started with Meditation: A Guide for Beginners 38

Understanding the Basics 38

Creating a Conducive Environment..38

Simple Techniques to Begin With 38

Overcoming Common Challenges 39

Textual Element: Starting Your Meditation Practice Checklist..............39

4.2 Mindfulness Meditation for Daily Pain Management......................40

Principles of Mindfulness..40

Daily Practices 40

Body Scan Meditation 40

The Role of Awareness..41

4.3 Guided Imagery: A Mental Escape from Fibromyalgia Pain............. 41

4.4 Deep Breathing Exercises to Soothe Pain Instantly 42

Breathing Techniques Basics 43

Step-by-step Guide 43

Integration into Daily Life..43

Long-term Benefits 43

4.5 Progressive Muscle Relaxation for Tension Relief 44

4.6 Creating a Personalized Meditation Routine for Long-term Benefits 45

Chapter 5 Advanced Meditation Techniques for Fibromyalgia Relief...........47

5.1 Moving Beyond Basics: Advanced Meditation Techniques 47

Introduction to Advanced Practices 47

Finding the Right Technique 47

Deepening the Practice..48

Mindfulness in Movement...48

5.2 Yoga Nidra for Deep Rest and Pain Relief   49

5.3 Loving-Kindness Meditation to Combat Loneliness 50

5.4 Zazen Practice: Sitting Meditation for Inner Peace 51

5.5 Tapping into the Power of Chakra Meditation........................... 53

5.6 Integrating Meditation with Daily Activities for Continuous Relief 55

Chapter 6 Lifestyle Modifications for Managing Fibromyalgia 56

- 6.1 The Impact of Sleep on Fibromyalgia and How to Improve It 56
  - The connection between sleep and pain 56
  - Sleep hygiene practices 57
  - Relaxation techniques for better sleep 57
  - When to seek professional help 57
  - Textual Element: Sleep Hygiene Checklist 57
- 6.2 Gentle Physical Exercises Tailored for Senior Women 58
- 6.3 The Role of Hydration and Nutrition in Pain Management 59
  - Nutritional Considerations for Fibromyalgia 60
  - Hydration and Its Effects on Pain 60
  - Creating a Balanced Diet 60
  - Supplements and Fibromyalgia 61
- 6.4 Environmental Adjustments for Better Living with Fibromyalgia 61
  - Creating a Fibro-Friendly Home 62
  - Ergonomic Considerations 62
  - Temperature and Clothing 62
  - Accessibility and Mobility Aids 62
- 6.5 The Power of a Strong Support System 63
  - Building a Support Network 63
  - Communicating Needs 63
  - Finding Community 64
  - The Role of Caregivers 64
- 6.6 Managing Stress Through Time Management and Prioritization 64

Chapter 7 Addressing Common Challenges and Objections 66
- 7.1 "I've Tried Everything": Overcoming Despair 66
  - Recognizing the Cycle of Despair 66
  - Reframing the Journey 66
  - Exploring Underutilized Options 66
  - The Power of Incremental Changes 67

Textual Element: Lifestyle Adjustment Checklist 67

7.2 Meditation Misconceptions: "It's Not for Me" 67

Debunking Meditation Myths 67

Showcasing Variety in Meditation 68

Personal Stories of Transformation   68

Guidance for Beginners... 69

7.3 Simplifying CBT: It is Easier Than You Think 69

Demystifying CBT 69

Self-administered CBT Techniques 69

Accessing CBT Resources... 70

Success with CBT... 70

7.4 Beyond Medication: Exploring Nonpharmacological Treatments 71

7.5 Tackling Isolation: Building Your Fibromyalgia Support Network 73

7.6 Coping with Flare-Ups: Practical Tips and Emotional Support 75

Chapter 8 Real Women, Real Success: Stories of Overcoming Fibromyalgia 76

Diverse Experiences, Unified Hope 76

Textual Element: Reflection Section... 77

Lessons Learned 77

The Role of Perseverance 77

Inspiration for Action 77

8.1 Setting and Achieving Personal Wellness Goals... 78

Goal-setting Principles 78

SMART Goals for Health 78

Celebrating Milestones 79

Adjusting Goals as Needed 79

8.2 The Role of Continuous Learning in Fibromyalgia Management 79

8.3 Embracing a New Normal: Life Beyond Fibromyalgia Pain... 81

8.4 Expanding Your Toolkit: When to Seek Additional Help 82

8.5 Celebrating Every Victory: Big or Small 84

Conclusion 85
References 86

Introduction

Every year, millions of senior women face the relentless challenge of fibromyalgia, a condition characterized by widespread pain, sleep disturbances, fatigue, and often emotional and mental distress. Despite its prevalence, the path to managing fibromyalgia pain can feel lonely and impossible. But what if I told you, it does not have to be this way?

My journey into the world of Cognitive Behavioral Therapy (CBT), meditation, and nutritional science was not by chance. It was born out of a deep-rooted passion to make a tangible difference in the lives of women seniors grappling with fibromyalgia. With years of research, practice, and seeing firsthand the transformative power of these tools, I have crafted this guide to extend a helping hand to those in need.

This book is more than just a collection of strategies; it is a mission to empower you to reclaim control over your life, reduce your pain, and enhance your overall well-being. Tailored specifically for senior women, every page and every chapter address your unique challenges. It needs in mind—making you feel understood, supported, and, most importantly, capable of overcoming the hurdles fibromyalgia presents.

Structured in three main parts, we dive deep into understanding fibromyalgia and how it affects your body and mind. From there, we explore the practical application of CBT and meditation—proven methods not just in theory but in real-life success stories of women who have triumphed over their fibromyalgia pain. The journey does not end there; we also tackle everyday challenges, offering you tools and techniques to navigate them with resilience and grace.

This guide's core belief is an integrated approach to managing fibromyalgia. We address the condition's physical and psychological aspects by integrating CBT, meditation, a balanced diet, and gentle exercises. This comprehensive strategy ensures that you are not just coping but thriving.

Throughout the book, you will find inspiring accounts from women seniors who, just like you, once felt at the mercy of their fibromyalgia pain but have since found relief and joy in life again. These stories are not just narratives; they are testaments to the effectiveness of the strategies discussed and a beacon of hope for what is possible.

As you turn each page, I encourage you to engage fully with the material, apply the strategies, and embark on your journey towards a life with reduced pain and enhanced quality of life. Consider this book not just a guide but a companion—one that walks with you, supports you, and cheers you every step of the way.

Thank you for entrusting me with your journey. Together, let us move towards a future where fibromyalgia no longer defines your days but instead becomes a manageable part of your life's rich tapestry.

The seven steps to reduce Fibromyalgia pain through CBT Therapy are

Step One- Diet and Hydration for fibromyalgia health (chapter 2)

Step Two- Pain Management Plan for fibromyalgia (chapter 2)

Step Three- Support System (chapters 3 and 8)

Step Four- Meditation and Deep Breathing (chapter 4 and 5)

Step Five- Getting Proper Rest (chapter 6)

Step Six- Easy Exercise for Fibromyalgia (chapter 6)

Step Seven- Incremental change and Goal setting (chapters 7 & 8).

Chapter 1

In the quiet of the early morning, when the world is just beginning to stir from its slumber, many women seniors find themselves wrestling with a relentless and invisible adversary: fibromyalgia. This condition, characterized by widespread musculoskeletal pain accompanied by fatigue, sleep, memory, and mood issues, remains one of the most perplexing puzzles within the medical community. Despite its prevalence, the journey to understanding, diagnosing, and managing fibromyalgia, especially in senior women, is fraught with complexities and challenges. Through a lens focused sharply on this demographic, this chapter seeks to shed light on the intricacies of fibromyalgia, unraveling its impact, the pivotal role of hormonal changes, and the unique hurdles faced by senior women.

Fibromyalgia in Women Seniors: A Detailed Overview
Epidemiology and Prevalence

Recent studies underscore the significant impact of fibromyalgia on the senior female population. According to research, fibromyalgia affects a more substantial proportion of women than men, with the disparity growing more pronounced with age. The prevalence among senior women is not just a statistic; it reflects the countless lives intricately woven with the daily realities of managing this condition. This data compels us to look beyond the numbers, recognizing each figure as a narrative of resilience and perseverance.

Understanding the Condition

Fibromyalgia, often shrouded in mystery, is a condition distinguished by chronic, widespread pain. Unlike other pain conditions that might be localized or linked to specific bodily injuries, fibromyalgia manifests as a pervasive discomfort, its origins deeply rooted in the complex interplay between neurological and physiological processes. The diagnosis, therefore, relies not on standard medical tests but on patient-reported symptoms and a thorough examination of pain distribution across the body. This diagnostic criterion sets fibromyalgia apart, emphasizing the subjective experience of pain and the need for a nuanced approach to treatment and management.

The Role of Hormones

The intersection of hormonal changes and fibromyalgia symptoms in senior women presents a compelling side of this condition's complexity. As women transition into menopause, fluctuating levels of estrogen and other hormones can worsen fibromyalgia symptoms. Estrogen is known to have an analgesic effect, potentially mitigating pain sensitivity. With the decline of estrogen during menopause, women may experience an intensification of fibromyalgia symptoms, underscoring the need for a tailored approach to managing the condition during this phase of life. This hormonal shift not only illuminates the biological underpinnings of fibromyalgia but also highlights the importance of considering the holistic health landscape of senior women in devising effective treatment strategies.

Unique Challenges

The unique challenges faced by senior women with fibromyalgia extend far beyond the physiological symptoms. Social isolation, a common issue among older people, can be particularly debilitating for those with chronic pain conditions. The invisibility of fibromyalgia worsens this isolation, as friends and family may struggle to understand and empathize with the unseen agony. Moreover, the age-related stigma surrounding pain and mobility issues can deter senior women from seeking help and advocating for their health needs. The convergence of ageism, gender bias, and the invisible nature of fibromyalgia creates a trifecta of challenges that senior women must navigate in their quest for relief and understanding.

Interactive Element: Reflecting on Your Experience

Reflect on a moment when your fibromyalgia symptoms felt particularly overwhelming. How did this affect your daily activities and interactions? Were there specific triggers you found, and how did you adapt to manage your symptoms during this time? This reflection can help you pinpoint patterns in your symptom flare-ups and be a valuable tool in developing personalized coping strategies.

In dissecting these components of fibromyalgia in senior women, we begin to unravel the layers of complexity that define this condition. The prevalence and impact statistics offer a stark glimpse into the widespread nature of fibromyalgia among senior women, challenging us to look beyond the numbers and acknowledge the individual stories of resilience. Understanding fibromyalgia requires us to delve deep into its symptoms and diagnostic criteria, recognizing the subjective nature of pain and the critical role of comprehensive assessment. The hormonal landscape of senior women provides a biological lens through which we can view the worsening of symptoms, emphasizing the need for personalized treatment approaches that consider the entirety of a woman's physiological changes. Lastly, the unique challenges faced by this demographic remind us of the importance of empathy, support, and advocacy in navigating the complexities of fibromyalgia. Through this detailed exploration, we lay the groundwork for a deeper understanding of fibromyalgia in senior women, paving the way for targeted strategies that address the nuanced needs of this population.

1.2 Debunking Myths: What Fibromyalgia Is and Is not

In a world where medical knowledge is at our fingertips yet often mired in layers of misinformation, fibromyalgia stands as a testament to the complex interplay between belief and reality. The myths surrounding this condition undermine its legitimacy and hinder those affected from looking for and receiving proper care. It is within this context that the imperative to dismantle these myths becomes clear, navigating through misconceptions to shed light on the tangible, physiological roots of fibromyalgia.

One pervasive myth posits that fibromyalgia is "all in the head," a misconception that trivializes the lived experiences of millions. This narrative insidiously suggests that the condition is a manifestation of psychological distress rather than a legitimate medical issue. Such viewpoints are not only scientifically unfounded but also contribute to the stigmatization of those diagnosed. The reality, underscored by a wealth of scientific research, reveals fibromyalgia as a disorder characterized by abnormalities in pain processing by the brain and nervous system. This evidence illustrates the physical basis of fibromyalgia, confirming the experiences of those who navigate its challenges daily.

Equally damaging is the myth that fibromyalgia is "just a woman's issue," implying a gendered bias that neglects the condition's presence across the spectrum of gender. While statistics show a higher prevalence among women, this narrative not only marginalizes men and non-binary individuals who have fibromyalgia but also perpetuates harmful stereotypes about pain and gender. Acknowledging fibromyalgia's impact beyond gender boundaries is crucial for fostering a more inclusive understanding and approach to care.

The battle against these myths is not merely academic; it carries profound implications for both those living with fibromyalgia and the broader societal perception of the condition. Misconceptions about fibromyalgia's legitimacy can lead to delays in diagnosis, with individuals often navigating a labyrinth of skepticism from both the medical community and their social circles. This skepticism can worsen the isolation felt by those with fibromyalgia, compounding the challenges they face.

In confronting these myths, the role of awareness becomes pivotal. Cultivating a deeper understanding of fibromyalgia among patients, healthcare providers, and the public is essential for dismantling stigma and promoting a more empathetic and practical approach to treatment. Awareness initiatives can illuminate the nuanced realities of fibromyalgia, highlighting the diversity of symptoms and the individuality of experiences. Such efforts can bridge gaps in understanding, fostering a communal approach to support and care.

The impact of misinformation on the treatment and belief of fibromyalgia cannot be overstated. Myths and stereotypes skew public belief and influence policy and healthcare practices. In instances where fibromyalgia is dismissed as a psychosomatic or exclusively female condition, the allocation of resources toward research, treatment, and support can be significantly affected. Countering misinformation with factual, research-backed information is paramount in advocating for the needs of those with fibromyalgia.

This advocacy extends into the realm of treatment, where understanding fibromyalgia's physical roots can catalyze the development of targeted therapies and interventions. Recognizing the condition's legitimacy paves the way for multidisciplinary treatment approaches that address both the physiological and psychological sides of fibromyalgia. Moreover, the drive towards awareness and understanding plays a critical role in shaping the narrative around fibromyalgia. Challenging and rectifying misconceptions shifts the dialogue from skepticism and dismissal to support and validation. This shift not only impacts those directly affected by fibromyalgia but also cultivates a more informed and empathetic society.

In navigating the myths and realities of fibromyalgia, the journey is not linear but rather a continuous process of education, advocacy, and support. Each step forward in debunking myths and disseminating accurate information strengthens the foundation for better understanding and care. For individuals with fibromyalgia, this journey is both personal and collective—a path walked together with allies, healthcare providers, and the wider community.

Dispelling myths and fostering awareness about fibromyalgia is more than an academic exercise; it is a vital component of improving the lives of those affected. Dedicated efforts to challenge misconceptions, validate experiences, and promote accurate understanding can transform the narrative surrounding fibromyalgia. This transformation not only benefits those living with the condition but also enriches our collective knowledge and empathy, moving us closer to a society where fibromyalgia is recognized, understood, and effectively managed.

1.3 The Invisible Battle: Understanding the Emotional Toll

In the realm of chronic conditions, fibromyalgia stands as a silent specter, its impacts echoing deeply within the confines of the mind and soul yet remaining invisible to the outside world. This invisibility cloaks sufferers in a veil of misunderstanding and often disbelief, exacerbating not only the physical pain they endure but also ushering in a cascade of emotional and mental health struggles. The battle against fibromyalgia is waged not just in the physical domain but in the psychological one, where feelings of isolation, frustration, and despair often take root.

For many, the first diagnosis of fibromyalgia brings with it a paradoxical mix of relief and trepidation. The diagnosis brings relief for the validation of their pain and suffering, trepidation for the journey ahead, fraught with the challenges of managing an often-misunderstood condition. The emotional toll of fibromyalgia is multifaceted, with anxiety and depression standing as somber landmarks in a landscape marred by chronic pain. Anxiety usually stems from the unpredictability of pain flare-ups, the constant apprehension of the next wave of discomfort, and the fear of being unable to fulfill roles and responsibilities. Depression, on the other hand, can take root in the feelings of isolation and the loss of one's former self, a shadow that grows longer with each passing day of relentless pain and fatigue.

The stigma surrounding invisible illnesses further compounds these emotional challenges. Unlike conditions with visible symptoms, people living with fibromyalgia navigate a world where their pain is often questioned or outright dismissed. This disbelief, whether faced in social circles or, regrettably, within the healthcare system, invalidates their experiences and drives many into the shadows, where they silently endure their suffering. The stigma attached to invisible illnesses not only hinders individuals from seeking the support they need but also perpetuates a cycle of isolation and mental health decline.

In confronting the emotional toll of fibromyalgia, the cultivation of effective coping strategies becomes paramount. The first step lies in the acknowledgment of the emotional and mental health impacts of the condition. Recognizing these as legitimate and integral aspects of the fibromyalgia experience allows for a more integrated approach to management—one that encompasses both the body and the mind. Mindfulness and meditation emerge as powerful tools in this regard, offering pathways to inner calm and helping to lessen the grip of anxiety and depression. These practices encourage a moment-by-moment awareness and acceptance of one's experiences, fostering a gentle understanding and compassion towards oneself.

Journaling offers immense therapeutic benefits. It provides a crucial outlet for expressing thoughts and emotions that might remain bottled up. Individuals can externalize their struggles by writing, making them more manageable and giving relief. Through writing, individuals can externalize their struggles, making them more manageable and affording a degree of relief. Additionally, engaging in support groups, whether online or in-person, mitigates the commonly felt isolation. These communities offer not just a space for shared understanding and empathy but also a repository of collective wisdom and coping strategies, invaluable for those navigating the fibromyalgia journey.

At the heart of these coping strategies lies the power of validation. The simple act of acknowledging the pain and struggles faced by those with fibromyalgia can have a profound impact. It is a recognition of their battle, an affirmation that their suffering is real and worthy of attention. Validation can come from various sources, including healthcare professionals, family, friends, or others who also experience fibromyalgia.

Each affirming gesture and acknowledgment acts as a balm, soothing the emotional wounds inflicted by the condition. It fosters a sense of community and belonging, breaking through the barriers of isolation and misunderstanding.

The emotional toll of fibromyalgia, while formidable, is not impossible. Through mindfulness, therapeutic expression, community support, and the seeking of validation, individuals can navigate the psychological landscape of their condition with increased resilience. These strategies, woven together, form a tapestry of coping mechanisms that not only address the physical manifestations of fibromyalgia but also honor the emotional and mental health challenges it presents. In doing so, they provide a beacon of hope, guiding sufferers toward a place of greater understanding, acceptance, and peace.

In this invisible battle, the victories may be quiet, and the Progress may be gradual. Still, each step taken toward emotional well-being marks a significant stride in the journey of managing fibromyalgia. With each breath, each word written, and each story shared, the weight of the condition lightens, making room for moments of joy, connection, and fulfillment amidst the challenges. Moving forward necessitates patience, compassion, and a steadfast dedication to self-care. It is essential to understand that the fight against fibromyalgia is not fought in isolation but with the support of a community that recognizes, listens to, and validates the experiences of those within it.

1.4 Fibromyalgia and Aging: Navigating the Double Challenge

Aging naturally introduces various bodily changes that can alleviate or worsen medical conditions. For women seniors grappling with fibromyalgia, the advancing years paint a complex picture, one where the brushstrokes of aging intersect with the chronic patterns of pain, fatigue, and cognitive fog characteristic of this condition. Understanding how fibromyalgia morphs in the face of aging is pivotal, not just for the sufferers but for the medical professionals aiding in their care.

Symptoms of fibromyalgia, though consistent in their impact, can shift in intensity as one grows older. The body's resilience, once a fortress against the relentless waves of discomfort, begins to wane, transforming minor flare-ups into prolonged battles. Pain, the hallmark of fibromyalgia, may find new residences in the body, areas previously untouched by its reach. Similarly, fatigue can evolve into a near-constant companion once manageable with rest and strategic pacing, overshadowing even the simplest daily tasks. Cognitive symptoms, too, often referred to as "fibro fog," can deepen, intersecting alarmingly with concerns over age-related mental decline.

This intricate dance between fibromyalgia and aging necessitates a recalibration of expectations. Women seniors must navigate this path with a sense of realism, understanding that the goalposts of management and relief may shift over time. This recalibration is not an admission of defeat but a strategic acknowledgment of the evolving nature of their condition. It calls for setting attainable goals that respect the body's current state, focusing on maintaining function and quality of life rather than pursuing the elusive promise of complete symptom eradication.

Lifestyle adjustments emerge as critical allies in this ongoing adaptation. Once perhaps a secondary consideration, nutrition now takes center stage, with a balanced diet as a cornerstone of symptom management. Foods rich in anti-inflammatory properties can offer respite from pain, while those high in antioxidants may combat the fatigue that often accompanies fibromyalgia. Exercise, too, must be approached with a new lens. Gone are the days of high-intensity workouts; in their place, gentle, low-impact activities such as walking, swimming, or tai chi become invaluable, their rhythms aligning with the body's capabilities while still fostering endurance and strength.

Sleep, an often-stormy aspect of fibromyalgia, demands a renewed focus.

Improving sleep hygiene through strategies like maintaining regular sleep schedules and creating a restful bedroom environment becomes crucial for alleviating the intensified symptoms caused by inadequate rest. Similarly, stress management techniques—be they through meditation, deep-breathing exercises, or engaging in hobbies—take on added importance, offering a buffer against the stress-pain cycle that can so easily ensnare those with fibromyalgia.

Preventative measures, grounded in the principle of early detection and intervention, hold the key to navigating the double challenge of fibromyalgia and aging. Routine medical evaluations become more than just a check-up; they are an opportunity for early identification of exacerbating symptoms or the emergence of new health concerns that could complicate fibromyalgia management. These evaluations also offer a platform for ongoing education for the patients and their caregivers, ensuring that all parties remain informed and proactive in addressing the condition's evolution.

Adaptations to the home environment, too, play a critical role in prevention. Modifications designed to reduce fall risks, ease mobility, and enhance overall safety can significantly impact a senior woman's ability to manage her fibromyalgia symptoms while maintaining independence. Such changes not only address the immediate concerns related to physical safety but also contribute to a sense of control and autonomy, factors crucial for emotional and mental well-being amid chronic pain.

At its core, navigating the intersection of fibromyalgia and aging is an exercise in balance, a delicate negotiation between acknowledging limitations and fostering resilience. It is a recognition that while fibromyalgia may indeed morph and evolve alongside the aging process, so too can the strategies employed to manage it. Through realistic goal setting, lifestyle adjustments, and proactive preventative measures, senior women with fibromyalgia can find a way to live with their condition, not merely endure it. This approach, rooted in understanding and adaptation, offers a path forward, one marked by hope, agency, and the pursuit of well-being amidst the complexities of aging with fibromyalgia.

1.5 Recognizing Fibromyalgia Symptoms Unique to Senior Women

In the landscape of senior women's health, fibromyalgia paints a picture that is both intricate and deeply personal. While the tapestry of symptoms woven by this condition shares common threads with the experiences of younger individuals, it includes patterns unique to the older demographic. For senior women, the manifestation of fibromyalgia symptoms often intertwines with the natural physiological changes occurring with age, creating a complex constellation of signs that demand both attention and understanding. Muscle stiffness, which greets many at dawn, is more severe in senior women. This stiffness, extending beyond the usual discomfort, can severely limit the initiation of daily activities, transforming mornings into a time of dread rather than renewal. Similarly, the widespread pain that is the hallmark of fibromyalgia often presents with increased intensity, its grip tightening around the shoulders, neck, and back, areas that also endure the most of age-related musculoskeletal wear.

Fatigue, a common symptom, becomes even more debilitating in senior women, its burden amplified by the body's diminished resilience to stress and illness. Unlike the tiredness experienced by younger individuals, this fatigue can persist even after ample rest, casting a shadow over the entire day's potential.

Moreover, cognitive symptoms, colloquially termed "fibro fog," manifest with heightened impact, blurring the lines between age-related mental decline and fibromyalgia-induced cognitive challenges. This fog, encompassing memory lapses and difficulties in concentration, can significantly disrupt the independence and self-sufficiency many senior women fiercely protect. The interplay between fibro fog and natural aging processes necessitates a vigilant approach to symptom management, ensuring that cognitive changes are accurately attributed and addressed.

The challenge, however, lies in recognizing these symptoms and differentiating them from those of other age-related conditions. Osteoarthritis, for instance, shares the symptom of joint stiffness with fibromyalgia but is localized to the joints and worsens with activity, unlike the pervasive stiffness of fibromyalgia, which often improves slightly with movement. Similarly, while both fibromyalgia and age-related sleep disturbances can lead to fatigue, the non-restorative sleep characteristic of fibromyalgia is distinct in its persistence despite sleep hygiene efforts.

This nuanced understanding is crucial to prevent misdiagnosis and accurately target treatments.

In navigating these complexities, the role of comprehensive care becomes paramount. Care for senior women with fibromyalgia must transcend the conventional boundaries of symptom management, embracing a comprehensive approach that addresses the multifaceted nature of the condition. Integrating physical, mental, and emotional health strategies, this approach acknowledges the interconnectedness of fibromyalgia symptoms with the individual's overall well-being. Physical therapy, tailored to enhance mobility and reduce stiffness without worsening pain, becomes a cornerstone of this care model. Concurrently, cognitive training exercises and strategies to cope with fibro fog support mental health, while counseling and support groups address the emotional and psychological toll of living with chronic pain.

Empowerment through knowledge stands as a critical pillar in navigating fibromyalgia in senior women. Understanding the unique symptomatology and its differentiation from other conditions equips individuals to advocate effectively for their health. This empowerment is not just about having conversations with healthcare providers; it is about engaging in those conversations from a place of informed confidence. It involves asking the right questions, seeking clarifications, and exploring all avenues of symptom management. Moreover, it empowers senior women to recognize the value of their own experiences and insights in managing fibromyalgia, fostering a collaborative partnership with their healthcare team rather than a passive acceptance of prescribed treatments.

By sharing their understanding and experiences, senior women with fibromyalgia can create a ripple effect, raising awareness about the condition and its unique impact on their demographic. This collective empowerment can lead to improved care models, increased research focus, and a higher quality of life for those affected.

Recognizing and addressing the symptoms of fibromyalgia unique to senior women requires a delicate balance between medical expertise and personal insight. It demands an informed and compassionate approach, acknowledging the individuality of each woman's experience while grounding care in the latest scientific understanding. Through this balanced approach, senior women can navigate the challenges of fibromyalgia with resilience, dignity, and fulfillment despite the presence of chronic pain.

1.6 The Importance of Early Detection and Management

In the labyrinth of chronic conditions that affect senior women, fibromyalgia often masquerades as a chameleon, its symptoms mimicking those of more familiar ailments and thereby eluding timely detection. The subtlety of its early signs usually results in a diagnostic odyssey, one fraught with missteps and missed opportunities for early intervention. It is within this context that vigilance becomes a beacon, guiding both individuals and their caregivers toward the early indicators that signal the presence of fibromyalgia. Among these harbingers are pervasive fatigue unalleviated by rest, a diffuse pain that defies localization, and a cognitive haze that clouds memory and concentration. Though seemingly innocuous when viewed in isolation, these symptoms collectively form a pattern that beckons further exploration.

The pursuit of an early diagnosis is not just seeking answers; it marks a critical juncture where the trajectory of fibromyalgia can change, guiding toward optimized management and improved quality of life. The merits of finding fibromyalgia in its nascent stages are manifold. Early diagnosis helps the implementation of targeted interventions that can significantly dampen the severity of symptoms, forestall the condition's progression, and mitigate the psychological toll associated with prolonged uncertainty. Furthermore, it opens the door to lifestyle modifications and therapeutic undertakings that lay the foundation for long-term symptom management. From dietary adjustments that cater to the body's heightened sensitivity to pain to exercise regimens that bolster physical resilience without worsening symptoms, the first stages post-diagnosis are pivotal in shaping a sustainable approach to living with fibromyalgia.

However, navigating the healthcare system in pursuit of a correct diagnosis demands more than just an awareness of potential symptoms; it causes a proactive and informed approach to communication with healthcare providers. This endeavor begins with articulating symptoms that transcend the mere recounting of discomforts, vividly depicting their impact on daily life. It involves not just listing the pains and fatigues but elucidating how these symptoms orchestrate a departure from normalcy, hindering activities once undertaken with ease. With a detailed symptom diary that chronicles pain episodes' frequency, intensity, and triggers, individuals can better advocate for themselves, transforming a potentially brief consultation into a thorough exploration of their condition. Moreover, preparing a list of questions before appointments ensures that conversations with healthcare providers are productive and informative, facilitating a collaborative partnership in the diagnostic process.

Upon securing a diagnosis of fibromyalgia, the journey that unfolds is one marked by adaptation and resilience. The initial steps post-diagnosis lay the foundation for building a life with fibromyalgia, accommodating the condition without letting it define them. During this phase, individuals actively adopt lifestyle adjustments to restore balance and minimize the impact of symptoms. Dietary changes, informed by a growing body of research on the interplay between nutrition and chronic pain, emerge as a cornerstone of this adaptive strategy, focusing on anti-inflammatory foods that soothe rather than exacerbate symptoms. Concurrently, integrating gentle physical activity into daily routines, tailored to the individual's capacity and preferences, fosters a sense of vitality, and combats the sedentary lifestyle that pain might otherwise impose.

Equally important in this nascent stage of fibromyalgia management is the cultivation of a support network, a tapestry of relationships that offers both emotional sustenance and practical assistance. Seeking out local or online support groups connects individuals with peers who share their experiences, creating a forum for exchanging advice, encouragement, and understanding. This sense of community, coupled with the support of family and friends, forms a bulwark against the chronic isolation conditions so often engender. Moreover, establishing a collaborative relationship with healthcare providers ensures that the management plan remains responsive to the evolving nature of fibromyalgia, adapting to the individual's changing needs and circumstances.

The early detection and management of fibromyalgia in senior women unfold as a multidimensional endeavor, one that interweaves vigilance, informed communication, and adaptive strategies. It is a process that acknowledges the complexity of the condition while affirming the possibility of a life marked not by limitation but by adaptation and resilience. Through early recognition, proactive healthcare engagement, and the implementation of tailored lifestyle adjustments, individuals can navigate the challenges of fibromyalgia with a sense of agency, crafting a pathway that honors both their needs and their aspirations.

Chapter 2 Holistic Approaches to Managing Fibromyalgia

In the tapestry of life, our diets are the threads that intertwine to form the fabric of our health. For women seniors navigating the complexities of fibromyalgia, understanding the nutritional intricacies can be akin to deciphering a code—where each food choice can either exacerbate the throes of pain or pave pathways to relief. This chapter delves into the symbiotic relationship between diet and fibromyalgia symptoms, exploring how strategic nutritional choices can serve as a keystone in managing this pervasive condition.

2.1 The Role of Diet in Managing Fibromyalgia Pain

Nutritional Impact on Symptoms

The adage "You are what you eat" echoes with profound resonance for those with fibromyalgia. Foods act as kindling to the flames of fibromyalgia symptoms, igniting flare-ups and intensifying pain. Conversely, a carefully curated diet can play a pivotal role in dampening the relentless ache, easing the fog that clouds the mind, and infusing the body with a semblance of energy previously thought lost. For instance, research underscores the inflammatory potential of processed sugars and saturated fats, which can amplify pain sensitivity and fatigue—a scenario all too familiar for people living with fibromyalgia. Conversely, omega-3 fatty acids found in fish like salmon and flaxseeds are celebrated for their anti-inflammatory prowess, offering a buffer against pain surges.

Dietary Changes for Relief

Navigating the dietary landscape requires a map that leads away from pain-inducing foods toward those that herald relief. Consider the Mediterranean diet a beacon of hope for many with fibromyalgia. Rich in fruits, vegetables, whole grains, and lean proteins, this diet champions foods that are not only anti-inflammatory but also rich in antioxidants, offering a double-edged sword against fibromyalgia symptoms. The emphasis on leafy greens, nuts, and seeds, alongside a modest dairy intake, provides a balanced approach to nutrition that supports overall health while specifically targeting fibromyalgia's grip on the body.

The Importance of Hydration

Hydration is a cornerstone of symptom management, often overshadowed by the quest for the right foods. Water, the most unassuming yet vital nutrient, plays a critical role in flushing out toxins that can contribute to symptom flare-ups. Moreover, adequate hydration ensures that nutrients are efficiently transported throughout the body, offering a steady energy supply, and facilitating the optimal functioning of every cell—a necessity in the battle against fatigue and cognitive fog. Encouraging a consistent intake of water throughout the day, coupled with the judicious use of herbal teas, can fortify the body's defenses against fibromyalgia's unpredictable onslaughts.

Personalized Nutrition Plans

The journey to finding the optimal diet for fibromyalgia is deeply personal, a puzzle where the pieces are as unique as the individuals assembling them. One size does not fit all, and the quest for dietary balance requires a tailored approach that considers personal tolerances, preferences, and nutritional needs. Engaging with a dietitian who understands the nuances of fibromyalgia can be transformative, offering guidance that illuminates the path to a diet that mitigates symptoms and enhances overall well-being. This partnership, rooted in understanding and adaptability, ensures that dietary strategies evolve with the individual's changing health landscape, offering a dynamic shield against fibromyalgia's erratic nature.

Textual Element: Your Personalized Fibromyalgia Diet Plan

Creating a personalized diet plan begins with observation. Start by keeping a food diary for two weeks, noting what you eat, when, and any symptoms you experience. Look for patterns—do certain foods trigger flare-ups? Are there meals that leave you feeling more energized or clear-headed?

Next, experiment with elimination. Based on your observations, gradually reduce, or eliminate foods you suspect may exacerbate your symptoms. Replace them with anti-inflammatory alternatives and note any changes.

Finally, consult with a healthcare professional or dietitian specializing in fibromyalgia. Share your food diary and observations. Together, create a balanced diet plan that addresses your specific needs and symptoms, ensuring it includes:
- A variety of fruits and vegetables are good for antioxidants and vitamins.
- Sources of omega-3 fatty acids for their anti-inflammatory properties.
- Whole grains and lean proteins to stabilize energy levels.
- Adequate hydration options tailored to your preferences.

Remember, managing fibromyalgia through diet is not about restrictive eating but about making informed choices that empower you to live with reduced pain and increased vitality.

2.2 Introduction to CBT: A Powerful Tool for Pain Management

Basics of Cognitive Behavioral Therapy

Cognitive Behavioral Therapy (CBT), a therapeutic modality grounded in the interplay between thoughts, feelings, and behaviors, emerges as a beacon for those navigating the turbulent waters of chronic pain. At its core, CBT operates on the principle that altering maladaptive thought patterns can catalyze a cascade of positive changes in emotional well-being and behavioral responses. This therapy, adaptable and person-centered, equips individuals with a toolkit for transforming the narrative around their pain, fostering a shift from a passive experience of suffering to an active engagement in symptom management. The methodology of CBT, structured yet flexible, unfolds through sessions where individuals learn to identify and challenge distortions in their perception of pain, gradually cultivating strategies that promote healthier coping mechanisms.

CBT for Fibromyalgia

In the context of fibromyalgia, a condition often cloaked in the ambiguity of invisible symptoms and fluctuating intensities, CBT offers a lifeline to senior women. This demographic, frequently at the nexus of age-related societal expectations and the isolating nature of chronic pain, finds in CBT a pathway to reclaiming agency over their bodies and narratives. Tailoring CBT to address the unique challenges posed by fibromyalgia involves a nuanced understanding of the condition's symptomatology—where pain is not merely a physical sensation, but a complex phenomenon influenced by psychological and emotional factors. Therapists' adept in this specialization guide individuals through the process of recognizing the triggers that exacerbate pain, the role of stress and anxiety in perpetuating symptom cycles, and the impact of lifestyle factors on their well-being. Through this guidance, senior women learn to implement practical coping strategies, from relaxation techniques and activity pacing to the establishment of realistic, self-affirming goals, crafting a life that accommodates fibromyalgia without being overshadowed by it.

Mind-Body Connection

The efficacy of CBT in managing fibromyalgia underscores the profound connection between the mind and body. This intricate and reciprocal relationship posits that the mind's perception of pain can influence the body's reaction and vice versa. For senior women with fibromyalgia, this connection often manifests in a feedback loop where pain triggers emotional distress, which in turn amplifies the perception of pain. CBT intervenes in this cycle by fostering mindfulness and self-awareness, encouraging a present-focused, non-judgmental appraisal of pain. This mindfulness, coupled with targeted behavioral interventions, helps to recalibrate the body's response to pain, diminishing its intensity and the associated emotional toll. Moreover, understanding the mind-body nexus empowers individuals to recognize the role of psychological stressors in their condition, paving the way for more holistic approaches to pain management that encompass both mental and physical health strategies.

Finding a CBT Practitioner

Embarking on the journey of CBT necessitates a partnership with a therapist who not only possesses the requisite expertise in cognitive-behavioral techniques but also exhibits a deep understanding of chronic pain management, particularly in the realm of fibromyalgia. Locating such a practitioner involves a multifaceted approach, starting with consultations with primary care providers or rheumatologists who can offer referrals to therapists specializing in fibromyalgia. Additionally, professional organizations and directories dedicated to CBT practitioners provide a platform for searching for therapists based on their focus areas and geographical location. Crucially, the selection process extends beyond credentials to encompass the therapeutic rapport—a mutual sense of understanding, respect, and compatibility that underpins the effectiveness of the therapy. Initial consultations offer an opportunity to gauge this rapport, allowing individuals to inquire about the therapist's experience with fibromyalgia, their approach to treatment, and their philosophy regarding the client-therapist dynamic. This discerning approach ensures that the chosen practitioner is qualified and aligned with the individual's needs, preferences, and therapy goals, setting the stage for a fruitful and empowering therapeutic experience.

In navigating the landscape of fibromyalgia, Cognitive Behavioral Therapy stands as a testament to the power of the mind in confronting and managing chronic pain. Its principles, grounded in the synergy between thought processes and physical sensations, offer a roadmap for senior women to traverse the complexities of their condition with resilience and hope. Through the strategic application of CBT, tailored to the nuances of fibromyalgia and bolstered by a supportive therapeutic partnership, individuals can cultivate a repertoire of coping strategies that transcend the bounds of traditional pain management. This journey, though challenging, illuminates the capacity for transformation inherent in the confluence of cognitive restructuring, behavioral adaptation, and an unwavering commitment to self-advocacy and well-being.

2.3 Meditation for Fibromyalgia: More Than Just Relaxation

Introduction to Meditation

In self-care and pain management, meditation emerges as a multifaceted practice that transcends the mere act of relaxation to touch upon more profound layers of healing and awareness. This ancient discipline, rooted in various cultural traditions, encompasses a spectrum of techniques, each designed to foster a unique state of mental clarity and tranquility. Meditation offers an array of pathways to inner peace, from mindfulness, which encourages acute awareness of the present moment, to focus attention, where the mind anchors to a specific object or thought. Another form, transcendental meditation, involves the repetition of a mantra to achieve a state of heightened awareness and rest. Each method, distinct in its approach, shares the common goal of harmonizing body and mind, creating a sanctuary of calm within the tumult of daily life.

Benefits for Fibromyalgia

For individuals grappling with fibromyalgia, meditation presents a beacon of hope, a non-pharmacological ally in the quest for symptom relief. The practice, by its stress-reducing properties, directly confronts one of fibromyalgia's notorious accomplices: stress. Chronic stress, a pervasive antagonist in the narrative of pain, finds its counterforce in meditation, which systematically lowers cortisol levels and soothes the sympathetic nervous system's hyperarousal. This biochemical shift alleviates stress and mitigates its physical manifestations, notably pain sensitivity. The role of meditation in enhancing sleep quality further underscores its therapeutic potential for people living with fibromyalgia. By cultivating a calm mind, individuals find it easier to transition into restful sleep, a precious commodity often disrupted by pain. Moreover, meditation's influence on pain perception is profound; fostering a detachment from pain sensations enables individuals to reinterpret their experience of pain, often leading to a notable decrease in its intensity.

Starting a Meditation Practice

Initiating a practice in meditation, particularly for those unacquainted with its disciplines, begins with small, deliberate steps. The initial focus should be consistency rather than duration; dedicating a few minutes daily to meditation can create a lasting habit. Selecting a quiet space, free from interruptions, allows for a deeper immersion into the practice. Comfort is paramount; whether seated, lying down, or walking, the chosen posture should facilitate rather than distract from concentration. The initial stages of meditation often involve a confrontation with a restless mind, a challenge best met with patience and gentle redirection. Acknowledging wandering thoughts without judgment and guiding the focus back to the breath or chosen to point of attention cultivates mindfulness, a skill that strengthens with practice. Establishing a routine by meditating daily cements this practice into daily life, transforming it from a task to a cherished refuge.

Resources for Guided Meditation

The journey into meditation, while deeply personal, need not be solitary. An abundance of resources exists to guide beginners through the intricacies of various practices, offering structured pathways to inner calm. Apps like Headspace and Calm stand out for their user-friendly interfaces and extensive guided meditation libraries tailored to different goals and experience levels. These digital platforms instruct and provide a framework for tracking Progress, encouraging sustained engagement with the practice. Websites dedicated to mindfulness and meditation, such as Mindful.org, offer articles, audio guides, and video tutorials, enriching the practitioner's understanding and technique. Books, too, serve as invaluable companions on this journey; titles like "Wherever You Go, There You Are" by Jon Kabat-Zinn and "The Miracle of Mindfulness" by Thich Nhat Hanh delve into the essence of mindfulness meditation, elucidating its principles with eloquence and accessibility. For those seeking a communal experience, local meditation groups and classes provide instruction and the support of a like-minded community, reinforcing the practice through shared experiences. These resources, each offering a unique perspective on the art of meditation, ensure that individuals embarking on this path have the tools and support necessary to weave meditation into their lives, transforming their relationship with fibromyalgia from one of struggle to one of harmonious coexistence.

2.4 Combining CBT and Meditation: A Synergistic Approach

In the realm of fibromyalgia management for senior women, the amalgamation of Cognitive Behavioral Therapy (CBT) and meditation emerges not as a mere conjunction of techniques but as a harmonious symphony of mind-body alignment. This fusion, rooted in the understanding that the physical sensations of pain and the mental narratives that frame them are inextricably linked, offers a dual approach to alleviating the multifaceted symptoms of fibromyalgia. Within this integrative framework, individuals discover the tools to navigate and transcend the limitations imposed by their condition.

The essence of combining CBT and meditation lies in their complementary nature. Where CBT provides the scaffolding for understanding and restructuring maladaptive thought patterns associated with pain, meditation offers a tranquil oasis from which one can observe these thoughts with detachment and compassion. This synergy fosters a profound shift in pain perception from an overwhelming force to a manageable aspect of one's experience. The cognitive strategies honed through CBT empower individuals to challenge and transform the distressing narratives surrounding their pain, while the mindfulness cultivated through meditation nurtures a state of serene acceptance. Together, these practices forge a resilient mindset equipped to face the ebbs and flows of fibromyalgia with grace and grit.

Case Studies and Success Stories

Senior women who have traversed the challenging terrain of fibromyalgia illuminate the potency of this combined approach, emerging with a renewed sense of agency over their well-being. Consider the story of Eleanor, a seventy-two-year-old who, after years of battling with fibromyalgia, found solace in the confluence of CBT and meditation. Eleanor's journey began with a skepticism towards meditation, a practice she initially dismissed as esoteric and unrelated to her physical pain. However, guided by a therapist specializing in chronic pain management, she embarked on a journey that transformed her relationship with fibromyalgia. Through CBT, Eleanor learned to identify and dismantle the negative thought patterns that amplified her pain, replacing them with affirmations of strength and resilience. Concurrently, daily meditation became a sanctuary for Eleanor to connect with her breath and cultivate a sense of peace amidst discomfort. Over time, this dual approach alleviated her symptoms and instilled in Eleanor a profound appreciation for the present moment, enriching her life in unexpected ways.

Developing a Personalized Plan

Crafting a personalized management plan that intertwines CBT and meditation begins with a commitment to openness and experimentation. The initial step involves an assessment of one's current coping mechanisms, discerning which strategies exacerbate pain and which provide relief. Armed with this insight, individuals can tailor their approach, selecting CBT techniques that resonate with their specific challenges and incorporating meditation practices that align with their preferences and lifestyles. Integrating these practices into daily routines necessitates flexibility, allowing for adjustments based on the evolving nature of fibromyalgia symptoms. Regular reflection on the effectiveness of these strategies, through journaling or discussions with a therapist, ensures that the plan remains dynamic and responsive to the individual's needs.

Overcoming Obstacles

The path to harmonizing CBT and meditation with the daily realities of living with fibromyalgia is not without its hurdles.

External pressures, fluctuating symptoms, and internal dialogues that foster doubt and resistance can challenge adherence to this combined approach. Overcoming these obstacles demands a multifaceted strategy that emphasizes self-compassion and the pursuit of support. Recognizing that setbacks are a natural component of Progress can alleviate the self-criticism that often accompanies lapses in practice. Furthermore, seeking the guidance of professionals who can navigate the intricacies of fibromyalgia management, alongside the solidarity of support groups, can bolster motivation and provide a reservoir of shared wisdom. The key to this process is cultivating patience, acknowledging that the benefits of combining CBT and meditation unfold over time and reveal their full impact through consistent practice and dedication.

In synthesizing CBT and meditation, senior women with fibromyalgia embark on a transformative journey. This journey, marked by the interplay of cognitive restructuring and mindful awareness, equips them to confront their pain with a newfound sense of empowerment. Through this integrative approach, the tumultuous seas of fibromyalgia become navigable, and the individuals who traverse them discover relief and a deeper connection to themselves and the world around them.

2.5 Tailoring Your Pain Management Plan: Tips and Tricks

In the nuanced world of fibromyalgia management for senior women, the profound significance of honing a personalized pain management plan cannot be overstated. This intricate process, akin to crafting a bespoke garment, demands an intimate understanding of one's physical and emotional landscape, where the feedback from one's body serves as the guiding light. Tuning into one's bodily cues transcends mere self-awareness, evolving into a dialogue where each sensation, each whisper of discomfort or ripple of energy, informs the choices that sculpt the contours of daily life. This deep listening, far from passive, is an active engagement with one is being, revealing insights that become the bedrock of a tailored approach to mitigating the effects of fibromyalgia.

Adapting daily activities to the ebb and flow of fibromyalgia symptoms requires a fluidity that mirrors the unpredictable nature of the condition itself. On days when the body sings a song of vitality, embracing more ambitious tasks aligns with the body's readiness to engage with the world. Conversely, recognizing the need for rest and gentler pursuits becomes paramount when the melody shifts to a sad tune of fatigue and pain. This dynamic calibration, though at times frustrating, cultivates a harmonious balance that honors the body's shifting capacities. It is a dance of give and take, where the rhythm is dictated not by external expectations but by the internal compass of well-being.

Incorporating gentle exercises into the fabric of this management plan introduces a thread of vitality that strengthens the overall tapestry when woven with care. Low-impact exercises such as tai chi, water aerobics, or walking emerge not as mere physical activities but as rituals of movement that celebrate the body's ability to engage with life despite fibromyalgia's constraints. These exercises, selected with discernment, offer a dual benefit—ameliorating symptoms while fortifying the body's resilience. The key lies in the gentle nature of these activities, which ensures that the pursuit of physical well-being does not devolve into a catalyst for flare-ups. Instead, it becomes a nurturing embrace, a reminder of the joy in movement and the subtle strength it builds within the fibrous tissues of one is being.

The quest for effective fibromyalgia management is not a solitary endeavor but a collective voyage that thrives on the support of a network woven from the threads of understanding and empathy. The scaffolding of this network, constructed from the pillars of healthcare providers, family, and friends, offers more than just a safety net—it provides a foundation of strength from which to confront fibromyalgia's challenges. Healthcare professionals, armed with expertise and insight, illuminate the path with medical guidance and therapeutic interventions.

Family and friends offer compassion and practical assistance, ensuring that the journey is not burdened by isolation. Their presence and willingness to listen and lend support transform the landscape of fibromyalgia management into one marked by connection and hope. Nurturing these relationships, inviting them into the inner sanctum of one's experience with fibromyalgia, fosters a shared journey where burdens are lightened, and victories are celebrated collectively.

This tailored approach to managing fibromyalgia, rooted in self-attunement, adaptability, and communal support, represents more than a strategy—it embodies a philosophy of living. It affirms the capacity to mold one's life around the challenges of fibromyalgia and to find a space for growth, joy, and fulfillment within the constraints. Through the meticulous crafting of this personalized plan, senior women with fibromyalgia navigate their condition with a sense of ownership and empowerment, charting a course through the turbulent waters with resilience and determination.

2.6 Understanding and Overcoming Common Treatment Barriers

In navigating the multifaceted landscape of fibromyalgia treatment, senior women often encounter a myriad of obstacles that can impede access to and adherence to effective management plans. These barriers, both personal and systemic, range from the labyrinthine complexities of healthcare systems and insurance frameworks to the internal battles waged against chronic pain and fatigue. Identifying these impediments is the initial step toward dismantling them, necessitating individual resolve and collective support.

Identifying Personal and Systemic Barriers

At the personal level, the very nature of fibromyalgia—with its unpredictable symptom patterns and varying intensity—poses a significant challenge. The fluctuating landscape of pain and fatigue can undermine motivation and the capacity to adhere to prescribed treatment regimens. Concurrently, systemic hurdles manifest in the navigation of healthcare systems that are often ill-equipped to address the unique needs of those with fibromyalgia, coupled with insurance protocols that may not fully cover the range of therapies deemed beneficial by medical professionals.

Strategies to Overcome Barriers

Tackling these barriers necessitates a multifaceted approach. For the individual, establishing a routine that accommodates the variable nature of fibromyalgia symptoms is crucial. Setting flexible goals that can be adjusted according to one's daily condition, thereby maintaining a course of treatment that is manageable and effective. Enhancing one's literacy regarding the intricacies of healthcare and insurance policies is pivotal on the systemic front. Armed with knowledge, whether negotiating with insurance companies to cover specific therapies or navigating healthcare systems to access multidisciplinary care teams.

The Role of Advocacy

Advocacy, both self-directed and communal, emerges as a powerful tool in confronting the barriers to effective fibromyalgia management. Cultivating the skills to advocate for oneself within the medical and insurance realms empowers individuals to secure the care and support they require. It contributes to a broader awareness of fibromyalgia's impact. Furthermore, joining forces with advocacy groups that champion the rights and needs of those with fibromyalgia amplifies this collective voice, potentially driving policy changes that facilitate better access to care and support services.

Utilizing Community Resources

The fabric of support woven by community resources, from online forums and support groups to local organizations dedicated to chronic pain, offers practical guidance and emotional solace. These platforms provide an invaluable exchange of information, from tips on managing symptoms and navigating bureaucratic hurdles to shared experiences that lessen the isolation often felt by those with fibromyalgia. Moreover, many of these groups engage in advocacy efforts to effect systemic changes that improve the treatment landscape for fibromyalgia. Engaging with these communities not only aids in overcoming personal and systemic barriers but also fosters a sense of belonging and collective strength among those affected.

As this chapter draws to a close, the essence of its message crystallizes into a beacon for those navigating the complexities of fibromyalgia treatment. Though fraught with obstacles, the journey is not a solitary endeavor, but a shared voyage buoyed by the twin sails of personal empowerment and community support.

The strategies outlined here, including recognizing, and addressing barriers to effective management and harnessing the power of advocacy and community resources, illuminate a clear path forward. Guided by resilience and bolstered by collective action, senior women with fibromyalgia can navigate these challenges, securing the care they deserve and fostering a landscape of understanding and support. This narrative, rich in challenges and triumphs, sets the stage for the subsequent exploration of the broader implications of living with fibromyalgia, beckoning us to continue this journey with an eye toward a future marked by compassion, understanding, and holistic care.

Chapter 3 Cognitive Behavioral Therapy (CBT) for Fibromyalgia Pain

The fabric of our thoughts weaves the tapestry of our reality, especially when chronic pain like fibromyalgia threads through the daily lives of senior women. Cognitive Behavioral Therapy (CBT) stands as a beacon, illuminating the path to reframe the mind's dialogue with pain, transforming the battleground into a place of strength and understanding. In this exploration, the efficacy of CBT unravels, revealing its potential to not only alleviate the physical manifestations of fibromyalgia but also to fortify the mind against the relentless waves of chronic pain.

3.1 CBT Explained: Changing Pain Through Mindset

Understanding Cognitive Distortions

Cognitive distortions, those skewed perspectives we hold about ourselves and the world, often intensify the experience of fibromyalgia pain. Like a lens that distorts the size and shape of an object, these distortions amplify our perceptions of pain, casting long shadows over our sense of well-being. "Catastrophizing," for instance, a distortion where we anticipate the worst possible outcome, can make a flare-up seem like an impossible crisis. Recognizing these distortions is the first step towards disarming their influence, allowing us to see our pain through a more transparent, balanced lens.

The Power of Thought Restructuring

Thought restructuring, a core component of CBT, empowers us to dismantle these harmful thought patterns and rebuild them into more constructive, realistic reflections. Imagine standing before a vast garden where weeds of negative thoughts about pain thrive. Restructuring thought teaches us to tend this garden meticulously, pulling out these weeds and planting seeds of positive, rational thoughts in their place. This process does not negate the existence of pain but changes how we interact with it, reducing its emotional and psychological impact.

CBT Techniques for Pain Management

CBT offers a toolkit brimming with techniques tailored for fibromyalgia pain management. An example is "graded exposure," which involves breaking down activities perceived as daunting due to fear of pain into manageable, incremental steps. This method not only facilitates physical activity but also rebuilds confidence shaken by fibromyalgia. Another technique, "behavioral activation," encourages the pursuit of activities that bring joy and fulfillment, countering the withdrawal and inactivity fibromyalgia induces. When practiced consistently, these strategies can significantly enhance the quality of life, even in chronic pain.

Building a CBT Toolkit

To further empower readers in integrating CBT into their fibromyalgia management regimen, we introduce a textual element:

Textual Element: Your Personal CBT Toolkit for Fibromyalgia

- **Pain Diary**: Keep a diary, noting when your pain occurs, its intensity, and the accompanying thoughts. This record will help you identify patterns and cognitive distortions linked to your pain experiences.
- **Thought Records**: Use thought records to challenge and change negative thoughts about pain. For each painful episode, please write down the idea, the evidence supporting and contradicting it, and a more balanced thought to replace it.
- **Relaxation Techniques**: Incorporate relaxation techniques such as deep breathing or progressive muscle relaxation into your daily routine to reduce stress and its amplification of pain.
- **Activity Scheduling**: Plan your week to include a balance of activities that need to be done and those you enjoy, avoiding overextending yourself. This balance is critical to managing fibromyalgia symptoms while engaging in fulfilling activities.

When utilized daily, this toolkit serves as a compass guiding toward a mindset where pain is not the commanding force. It fosters a relationship with fibromyalgia in which pain is acknowledged but does not overshadow the possibility of joy, fulfillment, and well-being. In the realm of CBT for fibromyalgia, the journey from recognizing cognitive distortions to actively restructuring thoughts and employing specific techniques marks a pivotal shift in managing chronic pain. This shift, rooted in the profound interconnection between mind and body, underscores the transformative potential of CBT. It is a testament to the resilience of the human spirit and the capacity to cultivate a life not defined by pain but enriched by a deeper understanding and mastery over the mind's landscape.

3.2 Identifying and Challenging Fibromyalgia-Related Negative Thoughts

Within the mindscape where fibromyalgia's whispers linger, a narrative steeped in negativity often takes hold, painting the condition in hues of despair and limitation. These narratives, though intangible, wield a tangible force, shaping perceptions and influencing the lived experience of pain. Recognizing these patterns is akin to mapping the contours of a shadow, acknowledging its presence while seeking the light that defines its edges.

Common refrains such as "I will never find relief" or "My pain defines me" echo through the corridors of thought, each step resonating with the impact of fibromyalgia on the sense of self and potential for happiness. The insidious nature of these thoughts lies not merely in their existence but in their ability to become self-fulfilling prophecies, reinforcing the cycle of pain and psychological distress.

Challenging these beliefs requires a delicate yet deliberate intervention, a process where introspection meets strategy. It begins with identifying these negative thoughts, holding them up to the light of scrutiny to reveal their distortions. This scrutiny involves questioning the evidence for each belief, dissecting its origins, and assessing its truthfulness. Such an exercise might reveal that the belief "My pain is unmanageable" is based on past experiences of ineffective treatment, ignoring instances of successful symptom management and moments of respite. The next step involves reframing these thoughts and crafting counter-narratives rooted in realism and resilience. For "I am powerless against my pain," a reframe might be "I possess tools and strategies to manage my pain effectively." This reframing does not dismiss the reality of pain but acknowledges the individual's agency and capacity to influence their experience.

Journaling emerges as a potent tool in this endeavor, serving as a mirror and a map. Individuals create a tangible record of their cognitive landscape by documenting thoughts, their triggers, and the emotions they evoke. This record, rich in insights, allows for tracking patterns over time, revealing the frequency of negative thoughts and their correlation with pain episodes. More importantly, it provides a canvas for practicing the art of reframing, enabling individuals to witness their progression from automatic negative thoughts to deliberate, balanced reflections. The act of writing offers a form of catharsis, a release from the mental confines fibromyalgia often imposes.

Yet, the journey through the terrain of negative thoughts and beliefs sometimes requires a guide, a professional who can expertly navigate the complexities of cognitive restructuring. Seeking support from a CBT therapist establishes a partnership where personalized strategies are developed, tailored to the individual's unique experience of fibromyalgia as well as their patterns of thought and belief.

In this therapeutic alliance, individuals can safely explore vulnerabilities and build new coping mechanisms step by cognitive step. The therapist's role extends beyond that of a navigator; they act as a mirror, reflecting the distorted beliefs in a new light, and as a mentor, teaching skills that empower the individual to become their therapist over time.

In this intricate dance of identifying, challenging, and reframing negative thoughts, the individual reclaims narrative control from fibromyalgia's grasp. This control does not imply the cessation of pain but represents a profound shift in how pain is perceived and experienced. It marks a departure from a path defined by fibromyalgia to one shaped by resilience, understanding, and hope. Here, the power of the mind is harnessed not as a vessel for suffering but as a tool for healing, illuminating the way forward with the light of positive, empowered thought.

3.3 Setting Realistic Goals and Celebrating Progress

Navigating the landscape of fibromyalgia, especially for senior women, necessitates a strategy where goal setting becomes an anchor amidst the flux of chronic pain. This approach, far from the rigid mandates of traditional goal setting, requires a fluidity that accommodates the unpredictable nature of fibromyalgia, crafting objectives that are as adaptive as they are achievable. In setting these goals, the emphasis leans heavily on the pragmatic—establishing benchmarks that resonate with one's current capabilities while gently pushing the boundaries of comfort and routine. In this context, goal setting is less about pursuing lofty aspirations and more about the incremental progression towards enhanced pain management and enriched quality of life. It is a delicate balance, where goals are neither so ambitious that they invite failure nor so modest that they yield no tangible sense of advancement.

The methodology for tracking Progress toward these goals demands precision and patience. It incorporates tools and metrics that reflect the multifaceted nature of fibromyalgia.

Pain scales, daily symptom and activity journals, and checklists of manageable tasks provide three lenses through which Progress can be actively monitored. This triangulation, far from a mere exercise in documentation, enables a nuanced understanding of how interventions—dietary adjustments, exercise routines, or cognitive strategies—influence symptoms over time. Such an approach quantifies the steps taken towards each goal and illuminates the often-subtle shifts in well-being, capturing the small victories that might otherwise go unnoticed. Recognizing these victories, however minor they may seem, is vital. These triumphs, small in isolation, collectively weave a narrative of Progress and resilience, reinforcing the value of the chosen path.

Adjusting goals as needed stands as a testament to the adaptive spirit required to live with fibromyalgia. It acknowledges that the condition, with its ebb and flow of symptoms, does not bend to the will of rigid plans. Instead, it demands a strategy as fluid as the symptoms, ready to evolve in response to new challenges and insights. This flexibility is not indicative of setbacks but of a realistic and responsive approach to managing a condition defined by its unpredictability. It might mean recalibrating the intensity of exercise on days when the body protests with pain or reshaping dietary goals when certain foods, once thought benign, reveal themselves as triggers. This ongoing revision of goals, far from a sign of failure, is an act of self-awareness and self-care, ensuring that the strategies employed align with the body's needs at any given moment.

Celebration, in the context of fibromyalgia management, becomes an act of defiance against the condition's attempt to overshadow one's achievements. It is a conscious decision to acknowledge every step forward to honor the effort and resilience that each step represents. These celebrations serve a dual purpose, whether they manifest as a quiet acknowledgment of a pain-free day or a shared moment of joy with loved ones. They elevate the spirit, infusing the journey with moments of lightness and happiness and fortifying the resolve to continue and persevere through the challenges. The act of celebrating Progress, regardless of its scale, fosters a mindset where optimism and gratitude take root, displacing the despair that chronic pain so often seeks to instill.

In this nuanced dance of setting realistic goals, tracking Progress, adjusting objectives, and celebrating achievements, the path through fibromyalgia becomes one marked by growth and adaptability. It is a path where each step, guided by pragmatic ambition and illuminated by moments of celebration, leads not just to the mitigation of symptoms but to a deeper engagement with life's potential despite chronic pain.

3.4 Coping Strategies for Fibromyalgia Flare-Ups

Flare-ups, those acute intensifications of fibromyalgia symptoms, unfold as unpredictable disruptions within the body, casting shadows of pain and fatigue that can eclipse the rhythm of daily life. These episodes, characterized by a sudden surge in symptom severity, serve as stark reminders of fibromyalgia's erratic nature. Triggers, as varied as the individuals they affect, range from physical stressors like an inadvertent overextension of activity to emotional upheavals or even shifts in the weather. The unpredictability of these triggers, coupled with their diverse origins, complicates the task of managing flare-ups, yet understanding their potential to provoke symptom intensification is the first step towards mitigating their impact.

In prevention, strategies that aim to minimize the frequency and intensity of flare-ups are as multifaceted as the condition itself. Among these is cultivating a lifestyle punctuated by balance and moderation. Regular, low-impact exercise fosters physical resilience, enhancing the body's ability to withstand the rigors of daily activities without crossing the threshold into overexertion. Concurrently, mindfulness practices and stress-reduction techniques, such as guided meditation or deep-breathing exercises, act as buffers against the emotional stressors capable of igniting flare-ups. Nutrition, too, plays a pivotal role; a diet rich in anti-inflammatory foods and devoid of potential irritants can stabilize the body's internal environment, making it less susceptible to the triggers of symptom intensification.

Despite the most meticulous preventive measures, flare-ups can and do occur, necessitating a repertoire of in-the-moment coping techniques designed to navigate these challenging episodes. Applying heat or cold, depending on individual preference and symptom manifestation, can offer immediate, albeit temporary, relief from pain. Heat, with its muscle-relaxing properties, can soothe stiffness and aches, while cold applications may reduce inflammation and numb more acute pain sensations. Distraction, a technique often underestimated in its effectiveness, provides a mental escape from the immediacy of discomfort; engaging in a captivating book, a film, or even a conversation can temporarily shift focus away from pain. Breathing techniques, particularly those emphasizing slow, deliberate breaths, can help modulate the body's pain response, offering a semblance of relief amidst the tumult of a flare-up.

Recovery from a flare-up, a process as individualized as the experience of fibromyalgia itself, requires patience and a gentle reacquaintance with one is routine. Prioritizing rest in the immediate aftermath of a flare-up allows the body to recuperate, restoring energy levels and mitigating residual pain. However, this convalescence period should not devolve into prolonged inactivity, as gentle movement can aid recovery, prevent stiffness, and promote circulation. The gradual reintroduction of activities, paced according to one's recovering capacities, ensures a return to normalcy that honors the body's limitations. This phase, critical in the flare-up cycle, underscores the importance of self-compassion and the recognition that recovery is not a race but a return journey to equilibrium.

Navigating fibromyalgia flare-ups, from understanding their triggers and implementing preventive strategies to managing their acute phase and fostering recovery, embodies the adaptive challenge of living with a chronic condition. It is a testament to the resilience and resourcefulness required not merely to endure the vicissitudes of fibromyalgia but to maintain a quality of life defined not by the presence of pain but by the capacity to adapt and thrive in its midst.

3.5 Enhancing Self-Efficacy in Managing Chronic Pain

The fabric of self-efficacy, particularly in fibromyalgia, is woven with threads of confidence, knowledge, supportive relationships, and dedicated self-care practices. This intricate weave forms a resilient barrier against the pervasive nature of chronic pain, offering individuals a foundation upon which to build a life not defined by their condition but enriched despite it. Self-efficacy, in its essence, embodies the belief in one's capability to exert control over one's functioning and events that affect one's life—a belief crucial for those navigating the unpredictable waters of fibromyalgia.

Building Confidence in Managing Fibromyalgia
Confidence grows from small victories and positive experiences in managing fibromyalgia. This confidence is not innate but a cultivated garden, requiring time, patience, and the right conditions to flourish. It begins with setting achievable, incremental goals—targets that, when met, reinforce the individual's belief in their ability to influence their pain and its impact on their life. Each goal achieved is a milestone and a beacon, illuminating the individual's capacity to navigate their condition successfully. This process of goal attainment, accompanied by a reflective appreciation of the effort and strategies employed, nurtures a growing confidence. This self-assurance strengthens with each step forward, no matter how small.

Role of Education and Skills Training
The empowerment derived from education and skills training adds a rich layer to the fabric of self-efficacy, reinforcing the foundation laid by confidence. In this context, knowledge acts as a shield, protecting against the uncertainties and fears that chronic pain breeds. By demystifying fibromyalgia—its triggers, symptom patterns, and management strategies—individuals arm themselves with the information necessary to make informed decisions about their care. Skills training, particularly in relaxation techniques, pain management strategies, and efficient communication with healthcare providers, equips individuals with practical tools to apply this knowledge. This combination of understanding and capability fosters a proactive stance towards fibromyalgia management, where individuals feel equipped to confront their condition with strategies that are both effective and personally suited to their needs.

Creating a Support System
Cultivating a robust support system introduces a dynamic element into the self-efficacy equation, offering a safety net and a source of strength. Supportive relationships, whether found in family, friends, healthcare professionals, or people living with fibromyalgia, provide more than just emotional comfort; they offer practical assistance, advice, and validation. This support network acts as a mirror, reflecting the individual's efforts and Progress and reinforcing their belief in their ability to manage their condition. Furthermore, these relationships serve as a sounding board, offering perspectives and strategies the individual may not have considered, thereby expanding their coping mechanisms. The act of sharing experiences, challenges, and victories within this supportive community not only alleviates the sense of isolation that chronic pain often engenders but also strengthens the individual's confidence in their capacity to navigate fibromyalgia.

Self-Care Practices
At the heart of enhancing self-efficacy lies the commitment to regular self-care practices, which acknowledges the importance of nurturing the body and mind. Self-care encompasses a spectrum of activities tailored to improve physical and emotional well-

being in fibromyalgia. These practices, ranging from mindful meditation and gentle exercise to adequate rest and nutritional mindfulness, form the daily rituals in which individuals honor their health and well-being. Significantly, self-care extends beyond the physical realm to include activities that foster joy, fulfillment, and relaxation, counteracting the stress and fatigue that fibromyalgia often brings. The consistent application of these self-care practices mitigates symptoms and reinforces the individual's sense of control and efficacy in managing their condition. It is through this dedicated self-nurturance that individuals find the strength to face fibromyalgia with resilience, crafting a life that, while acknowledging the presence of chronic pain, is not subsumed by it.

In the tapestry of managing fibromyalgia, enhancing self-efficacy emerges as a vital thread, intertwining confidence, knowledge, support, and self-care into a resilient whole. This fabric, rich in its complexity, offers individuals a foundation to stand as they navigate the challenges of chronic pain. It is a testament to the power of belief in one's capabilities, strength drawn from understanding and skills, comfort in supportive relationships, and the healing fostered by dedicated self-care. Through these elements, individuals with fibromyalgia cultivate not only the ability to manage their pain but also the capacity to thrive, embracing a life defined not by limitations but by possibilities and resilience.

3.6 Building Resilience Against Fibromyalgia Through CBT

In the landscape of chronic pain management, resilience emerges not merely as a trait but as a cultivated garden of strength, enabling those with fibromyalgia to navigate the complexities of their condition with a fortified spirit. In this context, resilience is the dynamic process of positive adaptation in the face of adversity; it is the ability to maintain or regain well-being despite continuous pain and fatigue. This concept transcends the mere endurance of suffering, embodying an active engagement with life's challenges and cultivating strategies that foster emotional and psychological robustness.

Cognitive Behavioral Therapy (CBT) acts as a loom where these threads are woven together, providing a structured method for cultivating resilience. Techniques grounded in CBT focus on the reconfiguration of thought patterns, the enhancement of coping skills, and the reinforcement of adaptive behaviors, all aimed at fostering a resilient mindset. One such technique involves the practice of cognitive reframing, a method where negative perceptions of pain are challenged and reinterpreted through a lens of positivity and possibility. This reframing alters the individual's internal dialogue about pain and influences their emotional response, shifting from a narrative of victimhood to empowerment.

Another resilience-building technique is the establishment of achievable challenges, tasks designed to stretch the individual's capabilities without overwhelming them. These challenges, whether social engagement, physical activity, or the pursuit of a hobby, provide grounds for resilience. Success in these endeavors, no matter how modest, bolsters self-confidence and reinforces the belief in one's ability to exert control over one's life despite the unpredictability of fibromyalgia. The incremental nature of these challenges ensures that each step forward is attainable and measurable, contributing to a cumulative sense of achievement and resilience.

The journey through fibromyalgia is marked by inevitable setbacks, moments where symptoms flare, and plans go awry. Within these setbacks lies a hidden curriculum, lessons in resilience that teach the individual to view these moments not as failures but as opportunities for growth and learning. The ability to extract wisdom from setbacks, to analyze what went wrong and why, and to adjust strategies accordingly transforms these experiences from sources of frustration into catalysts for development. This perspective fosters dynamic resilience that evolves in response to new challenges and insights. It is a resilience that acknowledges the reality of setbacks while refusing to be defined by them. At the core of resilience lies cultivating a hopeful, positive outlook on life that sees beyond the immediate confines of pain to the broader horizons of possibility.

This optimism is not a naive dismissal of the challenges of fibromyalgia but a purposeful decision to concentrate on achievable goals, celebrate potential, and discover joy in everyday moments. Techniques within CBT encourage this positive outlook through gratitude exercises, mindfulness practice, and engagement in activities that bring fulfillment and happiness. By focusing on the present moment and cultivating an appreciation for life's small pleasures, individuals learn to balance the scales between the challenges posed by fibromyalgia and the opportunities for enjoyment and meaning that life offers.

In weaving resilience into the fabric of fibromyalgia management, individuals tap into a wellspring of strength that enables them to confront their condition confidently and gracefully. This resilience, nurtured through CBT techniques, transforms the experience of living with fibromyalgia. It shifts the focus from pain and limitation to growth, learning, and the pursuit of well-being. Doing so enhances the individual's capacity to manage their condition and enriches their engagement with life.

In closing, the journey through fibromyalgia, guided by the principles of Cognitive Behavioral Therapy, reveals a landscape where resilience blossoms amidst the challenges of chronic pain. It is a journey that beckons not with promises of an easy path but with the assurance of strength, growth, and a deepened capacity for joy. As we continue to navigate the complexities of fibromyalgia, let us carry forward the lessons of resilience, the strategies for cultivating a hopeful outlook, and the commitment to transforming adversity into a wellspring of empowerment and well-being.

Chapter 4 Meditation Techniques for Pain Reduction

In the quiet moments between the cacophony of daily life and the whispers of the night, there lies a potent tool for healing—meditation. For women seniors grappling with the relentless grip of fibromyalgia, these moments of stillness are not merely pauses but opportunities for profound transformation. Within the serene embrace of meditation, the tumultuous relationship with chronic pain undergoes a subtle yet powerful metamorphosis, where the gentle touch of mindfulness softens the sharp edges of discomfort.

4.1 Getting Started with Meditation: A Guide for Beginners

Understanding the Basics

Meditation, often misconceived as an esoteric practice shrouded in mystique, unfolds as a simple, accessible exercise in awareness and focus. Its essence lies not in arcane rituals but in deliberately directing one's attention away from the chaotic stream of thoughts toward a chosen object, sound, movement, or even the breath itself. This conscious redirection cultivates a state of mental clarity and calmness, serving as a counterbalance to the stress and pain that fibromyalgia inflicts. Research underscores meditation's efficacy in not only reducing stress but also in managing chronic pain, offering a non-invasive, self-administered method for mitigating fibromyalgia symptoms.

Creating a Conducive Environment

Imagine a sanctuary, a personal haven where the outside world's demands momentarily fade into the background, and the focus shifts inward. Creating such a space, even within the confines of one's home, sets the stage for fruitful meditation practice.

You do not need a complex arrangement for this; a serene corner, cozy seating, and the gentle light of a lamp or the calming aroma of lavender can quickly turn a regular space into a meditative retreat. The key lies in consistency—returning to this designated space for meditation imbues it with a sense of sacredness and purpose, signaling to the mind that it is time to unwind and focus.

Simple Techniques to Begin With

Breath awareness is the cornerstone of meditation for beginners, a technique as natural as breathing. Focusing on the rhythm of inhalations and exhalations anchors the mind, drawing it away from distracting thoughts and toward the present moment. For those new to meditation, this practice can start with merely a few minutes daily, gradually increasing as comfort and concentration improve. Another simple technique involves silently repeating a personal word or phrase, serving as a focal point for the mind. These practices, simple in execution, open the door to the more profound benefits of meditation, making them ideal starting points for those embarking on their meditative journey.

Overcoming Common Challenges

Restlessness and distraction, the twin adversaries of meditation, often dissuade beginners from persisting with their practice. The mind, accustomed to constant stimulation, rebels against the calm, weaving narratives of discomfort or boredom. Addressing this challenge begins with acceptance—recognizing that distraction is a natural part of the meditation process. When the mind wanders, as it inevitably will, gently acknowledging this and returning focus to the breath or mantra cultivates patience and resilience. Over time, this process of noticing and redirecting hones the ability to maintain focus, transforming restlessness into serene attentiveness.

Textual Element: Starting Your Meditation Practice Checklist

- **Choose Your Meditation Spot**: Identify a quiet, comfortable space without interruptions.
- **Gather Essentials**: Consider a cushion or chair for seating, a blanket, and optional items like candles or incense to enhance the ambiance.
- **Set a Time**: Begin with short sessions, around 5-10 minutes, and gradually increase as you feel more at ease.
- **Select Your Focus**: Decide if you will concentrate on your breath, use a mantra, or follow another focusing technique.
- **Plan for Consistency**: Aim to meditate at the same time each day to establish a routine.
- **Address Distractions**: Keep a notepad nearby to jot down intrusive thoughts for later, freeing your mind to return to the practice.
- **Practice Patience**: Acknowledge that mastery comes with time and that each session is a step toward greater focus and calmness.

Incorporating these steps into the initial foray into meditation demystifies the practice, making it approachable and sustainable. As meditation becomes a regular part of daily life, the moments of stillness it brings evolve into a powerful ally against fibromyalgia's disruptions, offering not just relief but a pathway to a more centered, peaceful existence.

4.2 Mindfulness Meditation for Daily Pain Management

Principles of Mindfulness

At its core, mindfulness meditation unfurls as a practice rooted deeply in cultivating present-moment awareness, emphasizing an open, accepting, and non-judgmental stance towards one's experiences. This form of meditation beckons us to dwell in the immediacy of now, to observe the myriad sensations, thoughts, and emotions that flow through the consciousness without clinging or aversion. In the context of managing chronic pain such as fibromyalgia, mindfulness transforms the landscape of suffering, offering a lens through which pain is perceived not as an immutable force but as a series of fluctuating experiences. This shift in perception paves the way for a more compassionate and detached engagement with pain, where a broader awareness of the transient nature of all sensations tempers the raw intensity of discomfort.

Daily Practices

By weaving mindfulness into daily routines, one cultivates a steady presence that enriches every aspect of life, turning mundane tasks into opportunities for deepened self-awareness.

Each morning, start by setting intentions—a moment of quiet reflection where you envision the day ahead with a mindfulness objective, such as maintaining an openness to all experiences. You can integrate mindfulness into daily activities by savoring the flavors and textures of a meal or by practicing mindful walking, fully immersing in each step with awareness of your body's movements and sensations. When approached with conscious attention, even routine tasks transform into meditative practices, enriching the day with moments of presence and clarity.

Body Scan Meditation

One particularly effective technique for fostering mindfulness and addressing the physical manifestations of fibromyalgia is body scan meditation. This practice involves a gradual journey through the body, attentively noting sensations in each part without attempting to change or judge them. Start by finding a comfortable position, either seated or lying down, and close your eyes to turn the gaze inward. Begin at the feet, gently directing your focus to any sensations present—warmth, coolness, tingling, or even the absence of sensation. Slowly, with deliberate attention, move this focus up through the body, segment by segment, observing without attachment. This mindful exploration not only heightens body awareness but also reveals areas of tension and holding, allowing for a subtle and profound softening and release. The body scan is a relaxation technique and a bridge to a more intimate and compassionate relationship with one's physical self.

The Role of Awareness
Central to mindfulness meditation is cultivating awareness, particularly about understanding pain triggers and the body's nuanced responses to stress. Through consistent mindfulness practice, one develops an acute sensitivity to the precursors of pain flare-ups and stress, noticing the subtle shifts in bodily sensations or thought patterns that herald discomfort. This heightened awareness allows for early intervention, employing mindfulness techniques to mitigate the intensity of pain or employing coping strategies before stress escalates into a physiological response. Moreover, mindfulness fosters a deeper understanding of the interconnectedness of mind and body, illuminating how psychological stress, when unchecked, can amplify physical pain. With this knowledge, individuals are better positioned to manage their fibromyalgia, applying mindfulness not only as a reactive tool in moments of acute pain but as a proactive strategy in daily stress management.

In the gentle embrace of mindfulness meditation, individuals find refuge from the tumult of chronic pain and a transformative practice that reshapes their relationship with discomfort. This practice, with its roots in ancient traditions yet applicability in the modern struggle against fibromyalgia, is a testament to the enduring power of awareness, acceptance, and present-moment engagement. Mindfulness does not erase the experience of pain. Yet, mindfulness profoundly alters the suffering it engenders, shifting the focus from fibromyalgia's dominance to the richness of each lived moment.

4.3 Guided Imagery: A Mental Escape from Fibromyalgia Pain

Within the realm of meditative practices, guided imagery emerges as a beacon for those navigating the tumultuous waters of fibromyalgia. This technique, rooted in the principle of mind-body connectivity, utilizes the power of the imagination to evoke sensory experiences that can lead to tangible changes in physical and emotional states. The essence of guided imagery lies in its ability to transport the individual to a place of peace and comfort, far removed from the present reality of pain and discomfort, through visualization. It operates on the understanding that the mind can influence the body's response to pain, offering a respite that, while momentarily abstract, has concrete effects on wellbeing.

Creating personal imagery tailored to one's specific pain points begins with an inward journey, a deep dive into the self where the landscape of one's pain is acknowledged and embraced. It requires an attunement to the body's signals and an openness to explore the nuances of personal pain experiences. From this exploration, imagery can be crafted—visualizing a warm, gentle wave washing over areas of tension or imagining a cool breeze soothing inflamed joints. The key is specificity; the more detailed and personal the imagery, the more potent its impact. This visualization is not mere fancy but a deliberate construction of a mental sanctuary where pain is acknowledged but stripped of its power to dominate.

Turning to resources for guided imagery scripts and recordings can significantly enhance this practice, offering structured pathways to navigate one's inner world. Numerous online platforms provide access to many guided imagery sessions, ranging from general relaxation themes to those specifically designed for pain management. Libraries and bookstores, too, are treasure troves of audio recordings and written scripts that guide listeners through vivid, immersive experiences designed to reduce stress and alleviate pain. These resources act as compasses, directing the individual through the landscapes of their mind, ensuring that the journey is both fruitful and aligned with their healing objectives.

The efficacy of guided imagery in mitigating the symptoms of fibromyalgia is not merely anecdotal but is grounded in a growing body of research. Studies have significantly reduced pain intensity and stress levels among those who regularly engage in guided imagery practices. This reduction is attributed to the technique's ability to elicit the relaxation response, a physiological state opposite to stress, where heart rate slows, blood pressure drops, and muscles relax. Furthermore, guided imagery has been shown to positively affect the immune system and enhance sleep quality, which is crucial for individuals with fibromyalgia. The mechanism behind these benefits lies in the technique's ability to shift focus away from pain, reducing the brain's pain signals and altering pain perception. This shift not only diminishes the immediate experience of pain but also contributes to a long-term reconditioning of the body's response to fibromyalgia symptoms.

Incorporating guided imagery into one's pain management strategy offers a form of liberation, a way to reclaim control over one's body and experience pain. It invites a collaboration between imagination and physiology, where each guided visualization acts as a bridge to improved health and wellbeing. Through this practice, individuals find not only relief from the physical symptoms of fibromyalgia but also a renewed sense of hope and empowerment. Guided imagery, with its blend of creativity, relaxation, and healing, stands as a testament to the resilience of the human spirit and the untapped potential within each person to influence their journey with fibromyalgia.

4.4 Deep Breathing Exercises to Soothe Pain Instantly

In the tapestry of strategies woven to combat the pervasive discomfort wrought by fibromyalgia, deep breathing exercises emerge as threads of simplicity and efficacy. These practices, rooted in the primal act of respiration, offer a bridge to immediate and profound tranquility and pain alleviation. The essence of deep breathing lies in its capacity to signal the body's relaxation response, a physiological shift away from the stress-induced fight-or-flight state towards one of rest and repair. This transition, marked by a slowing heart rate and a decrease in blood pressure, sets the stage for a reduction in muscle tension and, consequently, a decrease in pain perception.

Breathing Techniques Basics

The foundation of deep breathing exercises rests on the deliberate slowing and deepening of breaths, a conscious counter to the shallow, rapid breathing that stress and pain often induce. This process involves diaphragmatic breathing, which focuses on expanding the lungs and engaging the diaphragm, rather than the chest, to draw in air. Such a method enriches the body with oxygen, enhancing cellular function and promoting a sense of physical and mental calm. The initiation of this practice requires only a moment's pause, a shift in attention to the rhythm of one's breath, and the intent to breathe deeply and fully. This simple act, accessible at any time and place, becomes a powerful tool in the modulation of pain and fostering a serene mental state.

Step-by-step Guide

To embark on deep breathing, one might begin by finding a position of comfort, whether seated with feet flat on the ground and spine straight or lying down with hands resting gently on the abdomen. The first step is to exhale completely, clearing the airways that prepare the body for deep inhalation. Following this, a slow, measured inhale through the nose fills the lungs, focusing on the expansion of the abdomen rather than the chest. This inhalation should be held for a brief count, allowing the body to absorb the oxygen before a gradual exhalation through the mouth ensues, releasing tension and stress with the departing breath. Repeating this cycle for several minutes creates a rhythm, a dance of breath that gently coaxes the body into a state of relaxation and pain relief.

Integration into Daily Life

The beauty of deep breathing exercises lies in their versatility and ease of integration into daily life. Moments ideally suited for this practice abound, from the quiet reflection of morning's first light to the lulls in activity that punctuate the day. Instances of waiting, whether in line at the grocery store or during the brief pauses of household chores, transform into opportunities for deep breathing, turning potential frustration into moments of serenity. The onset of pain or stress signals a pivotal moment to apply deep breathing exercises, proactively managing pain before discomfort escalates. Furthermore, the transition to sleep, often a challenge for those with fibromyalgia, becomes a prime time for deep breathing, promoting relaxation, and easing the journey to restfulness.

Long-term Benefits

While the immediate effects of deep breathing exercises on pain and tension are palpable, the long-term benefits accrue with consistency and dedication to practice. Over time, the regular invocation of the body's relaxation response through deep breathing reduces the overall intensity and frequency of fibromyalgia pain. This sustained practice not only diminishes the physiological impact of stress on the body but also enhances emotional resilience, equipping individuals with a robust tool for navigating the challenges of chronic pain. Moreover, the cultivation of deep breathing as a reflexive response to stress and discomfort promotes a proactive stance towards health, one in which pain management is interwoven with daily activities, empowering individuals to maintain a sense of control and wellbeing amidst the unpredictability of fibromyalgia.

In the realm of fibromyalgia management, deep breathing exercises stand as a testament to the power of simple, accessible practices in modulating pain and enhancing quality of life. Through the deliberate focus on breath, individuals find a pathway to immediate relief and long-term improvement, a journey marked not by complexity but by the return to a fundamental aspect of life—breath.

4.5 Progressive Muscle Relaxation for Tension Relief

In the complex landscape of pain that fibromyalgia creates, muscle tension often acts both as a symptom and an exacerbator, compounding discomfort and restricting the ease of daily movements. This tension, a silent architect of distress, weaves its threads tightly around muscles, offering a constant reminder of the condition's presence. The interplay between stress and pain is not merely coincidental but deeply intertwined, where each increment in muscle tightness seems to amplify the fibromyalgia pain experience, setting a cycle of discomfort that challenges both body and spirit.

Progressive Muscle Relaxation (PMR) is a beacon of relief in this cycle, a systematic practice designed to teach the body new narratives of relaxation and ease. The essence of PMR lies in its simplicity—an intentional contraction followed by a deliberate release of muscles throughout the body. This process educates the nervous system in the art of letting go. This technique, grounded in the principle of contrast, allows one to deeply appreciate the state of relaxation by first heightening awareness of tension. The benefits extend beyond the immediate release of muscle tightness; they ripple outward, reducing overall stress levels, diminishing pain sensations, and enhancing sleep quality, all of which are crucial for those living with fibromyalgia.

Embarking on a PMR session invites an intimate dialogue with one's body, a step-by-step exploration of tension and release that begins with the breath. A deep inhalation sets the stage, signaling readiness, while a slow exhalation ushers in relaxation, a prelude to the focused practice that follows. The journey commences at the extremities, often the feet, where muscles are tensed with the intention for a brief span, five to ten seconds, then released on an exhale, allowing the sensation of relaxation to wash over the area. This systematic progression moves upward, from the feet to the calves, thighs, abdomen, and so on, each step a deliberate act of release. Attention is lavished on commonly affected areas by fibromyalgia, where muscles might harbor deeper reservoirs of tension. Here, the contrast between tension and relaxation becomes most pronounced, offering vivid insights into the body's capacity for ease.

Integrating PMR into one's daily routine emerges as an act of self-care, a dedicated effort to reclaim moments of peace from the grip of fibromyalgia. For optimal benefits, consistency is vital; engaging in PMR daily, especially during periods of heightened stress or before sleep, can significantly alter the body's response to pain. Initially, audio recordings or instructions might guide the sessions, supporting the rhythm of contraction and release. However, as familiarity with the practice deepens, PMR becomes an intuitive ritual, easily adapted to the rhythms of the day, offering a flexible tool for managing pain and tension.

In the narrative of fibromyalgia management, PMR offers a chapter of hope, a testament to the body's resilience and capacity for relaxation. Through regular engagement with this practice, individuals learn not only to alleviate physical tension but also to cultivate a mental space of calm, a sanctuary from the storms of chronic pain. With its profound simplicity and benefits, this technique is a vital component of a holistic approach to managing fibromyalgia, a practice that soothes, restores, and empowers.

4.6 Creating a Personalized Meditation Routine for Long-term Benefits

The intricate nuances of fibromyalgia, a condition that paints every individual's experience with its unique shade of discomfort, necessitates a meditation routine that is not one-size-fits-all but tailored. This personalization begins with carefully examining one's pain landscape, lifestyle rhythms, and personal inclinations. Assessing these elements allows crafting a meditation practice that resonates deeply, offering a temporary respite from pain and a lasting sanctuary of calm.

When considering specific pain points, it becomes clear that the physical and emotional facets of fibromyalgia demand a diverse arsenal of meditation strategies.

For some, guided imagery that transports the mind to a serene place may best alleviate sharp, piercing pain. In contrast, others may find that progressive muscle relaxation, which releases subtle tension, more effectively eases diffuse, aching discomfort. Lifestyle, with its myriad duties and pace, further influences this customization. A busy individual might find shorter, more focused breathing exercises woven into the fabric of their day more practical than longer mindfulness meditation sessions, which may fit seamlessly into the routines of those with more flexible schedules.

The confluence of these meditation techniques into a cohesive, effective routine invites creativity and experimentation. It might involve starting the day with a brief mindfulness practice to set a tone of presence and calm, using deep breathing exercises as a quick tool for managing stress and pain spikes throughout the day, and ending with a guided imagery session or progressive muscle relaxation before sleep to ensure restfulness. This blending not only maximizes the benefits by addressing various aspects of fibromyalgia but also keeps the practice engaging and adaptable to changing needs and preferences.

Setting achievable goals within this personalized routine encourages consistency, a cornerstone of reaping meditation's long-term benefits. Goals range from the simplicity of meditating for five minutes every morning to the more ambitious aim of integrating mindfulness into every activity. The key to these goals lies in their realism and flexibility; they should stretch the individual's capabilities without straining them, allowing for growth in the practice without discouragement. Tracking progress through a meditation journal or app is a motivator and a reflective tool, revealing patterns and preferences that can guide further routine customization.

Flexibility in adjusting this routine over time ensures that it remains responsive to the evolving nature of fibromyalgia and the individual's journey with it. Just as the condition's symptoms may fluctuate, so too might the effectiveness of specific meditation techniques. Regularly reassessing the routine becomes an exercise in mindfulness, an attunement to the body's signals and the mind's needs. Adjustments might include:

- Exploring new meditation forms.
- Altering the duration of sessions.
- Shifting the focus of practices to address emerging challenges or capitalize on newfound strengths.

This dynamic approach fosters a meditation practice that is not static but living, growing in depth and breadth alongside the individual.

In weaving this personalized tapestry of meditation, individuals with fibromyalgia forge a powerful tool for managing their symptoms, enhancing their quality of life in a manner that is deeply personal and profoundly effective. The routine they create becomes more than a series of exercises; it evolves into a rhythm of self-care that resonates through every facet of their lives, bringing ease where there is discomfort, calm where there is turbulence, and strength where there is vulnerability.

As we close this exploration of creating a personalized meditation routine, the journey with fibromyalgia is deeply personal yet universally shared among those it touches. The strategies discussed here — assessing individual needs, combining diverse techniques, setting realistic goals, and remaining flexible — form a roadmap for navigating this journey. They underscore the power of meditation not just as a tool for managing symptoms but as a pathway to a more centered, peaceful existence, even in the face of chronic pain. This chapter is one step in a broader voyage toward wellbeing, continuing with resilience, innovation, and hope.

Chapter 5 Advanced Meditation Techniques for Fibromyalgia Relief

In the quiet predawn hours, when the world holds its breath, awaiting the sunrise, a woman finds solace in her meditation practice. This time, reserved for her alone, becomes a sacred space where she can confront the challenges posed by fibromyalgia. In these moments of stillness, she discovers the profound impact of advanced meditation techniques on her pain and wellbeing. From the gentle flow of mindful movement to the structured discipline of focused breathing, these practices offer more than symptom relief; they provide a pathway to deeper self-awareness and resilience.

5.1 Moving Beyond Basics: Advanced Meditation Techniques

Introduction to Advanced Practices

Advanced meditation practices, stepping beyond the foundational techniques of mindful breathing and body scans, open a more profound, nuanced exploration into the mind-body connection. These practices, ranging from dynamic meditation forms like walking meditation to disciplined approaches such as Zazen, demand time, dedication, and openness to delve into the subtleties of one's inner landscape. The rewards, however, are immeasurable, offering enhanced control over fibromyalgia symptoms, a profound sense of inner peace, and an enriched understanding of the self.

The potential benefits of these advanced techniques extend far beyond immediate symptom relief. Regular practitioners report reductions in pain and stress and improvements in sleep quality, emotional regulation, and overall life satisfaction. These outcomes reflect the physical adjustments that meditation can foster and the transformative psychological shifts that accompany deep, sustained practice.

Finding the Right Technique

Selecting an advanced meditation technique that aligns with personal needs and lifestyle is akin to choosing the right instrument in an orchestra. Each has its unique tone, resonance, and role in creating harmony. For someone seeking to integrate meditation seamlessly into a busy daily routine, walking meditation can turn a simple commute into a profound mindfulness practice. Conversely, for those who find solace in structure and stillness, the disciplined practice of Zazen offers a grounding counterpoint to the fluctuating symptoms of fibromyalgia.

When exploring these options, attending workshops or retreats can provide invaluable insights. These immersive experiences allow for direct engagement with different meditation styles under the guidance of experienced practitioners. Moreover, they offer a community of fellow meditators, providing support and inspiration. For those unable to attend in person, online courses and guided sessions offer a flexible alternative, making advanced meditation practices accessible regardless of location or schedule.

Deepening the Practice

Deepening one's meditation practice is not about allocating more hours to sitting in silence; it is about cultivating a quality of attention and intention in every moment. Techniques like mindful journaling, where reflections on daily meditations are recorded, can reveal patterns, insights, and areas for growth. This textual element serves as a mirror, reflecting the evolving relationship with meditation and its impact on fibromyalgia management.

Another effective strategy for deepening practice involves setting specific, achievable goals. These include increasing the duration of each session, incorporating mindfulness into additional daily activities, or mastering a particular meditation technique. Achieving these goals not only fosters a sense of accomplishment but also solidifies the role of meditation in managing fibromyalgia.

Mindfulness in Movement

Integrating mindfulness into movement transforms ordinary physical activities into rich opportunities for meditation. Practices like walking meditation or Tai Chi blend the physical benefits of gentle exercise with meditation's mental clarity and focus. In walking meditation, each step becomes an act of mindfulness, drawing attention to the sensations of movement, the rhythm of the breath, and the experience of the present moment. With its fluid, deliberate movements, Tai Chi offers a similar blend of physical and mental engagement, promoting balance, flexibility, and tranquility.

This integration of mindfulness and movement enhances the physical management of fibromyalgia symptoms and cultivates a deep, enduring sense of presence and awareness. It turns moving through the world into a continuous meditation, where every step and breath becomes a testament to the power of mindful presence.

In navigating the advanced landscapes of meditation, individuals with fibromyalgia venture beyond mere symptom management. They explore the self deeply, discovering relief from pain and a more profound sense of peace, resilience, and connection to the world around them. These advanced practices offer techniques and a way of living imbued with mindfulness, compassion, and a profound engagement with each moment.

5.2 Yoga Nidra for Deep Rest and Pain Relief

Yoga Nidra, often called yogic sleep, presents an intriguing paradox: deep rest coupled with full consciousness. This ancient practice, rooted in the traditions of Tantra, offers a systematic method of inducing complete physical, mental, and emotional relaxation. Unlike the cessation of sleep-related activity, Yoga Nidra facilitates a dynamic journey into the subconscious and superconscious realms, unlocking the potential for healing and self-discovery. Its relevance to pain management, particularly for those battling the complexities of fibromyalgia, lies in its capacity to bridge the gap between the conscious mind and the physical body, allowing for profound levels of relaxation and pain relief.

Engaging in yoga Nidra is to step into a world where the boundaries of awareness dissolve, inviting a deep sense of tranquility and detachment from physical discomfort. The practice begins with preparing the physical environment and the body; a quiet, dimly lit space free from interruptions complements the supine position adopted by the practitioner, supported by cushions or blankets for comfort. This initial stage, akin to setting the stage for a play, ensures that external conditions support the inward journey that Yoga Nidra promises.

Progressing from this preparatory phase, the practitioner embarks on a structured sequence of steps designed to guide the consciousness away from the external world and into the depths of the inner self. Starting with a Sankalpa, or resolve—a short, positive statement of intent—the individual plants the seeds for transformation and healing. Following the Sankalpa, a systematic rotation of consciousness through the body ensues, with attention directed to various parts, from the tips of the toes to the crown of the head. This meticulous scan heightens body awareness and diffuses physical tension, laying the groundwork for more profound relaxation.

Breath awareness and visualization techniques further deepen the relaxation, with the breath bridging the physical and subtle bodies. Guided imagery, a staple of Yoga Nidra, transports the practitioner to serene landscapes or situations, invoking sensory experiences promoting peace and wellbeing. This immersive visualization distracts the mind from physical discomfort and taps into the subconscious, eliciting positive emotional and physiological responses.

For those grappling with fibromyalgia, the benefits of Yoga Nidra extend beyond the immediate experience of relaxation. Regular practice has been shown to enhance sleep quality, a critical factor in managing fibromyalgia symptoms. The deep rest afforded by Yoga Nidra mimics the restorative stages of sleep, offering a reprieve from the cycle of pain and insomnia that often accompanies fibromyalgia. Additionally, the practice significantly reduces stress levels, with the relaxation response counteracting the body's stress-induced reactions, thereby diminishing pain intensity. This dual effect—improved sleep and reduced stress—contributes to a noticeable decrease in the overall impact of fibromyalgia on daily life.

A wealth of resources is available to facilitate access to the profound benefits of Yoga Nidra, from guided sessions led by experienced practitioners to recordings and scripts that allow for self-guided practice. Many online platforms and wellness centers offer Yoga Nidra classes explicitly tailored for pain relief, providing support and guidance for those new to the practice. Books and audio resources, carefully curated to include a variety of Yoga Nidra scripts, enable practitioners to explore different facets of the practice, ensuring that each session remains fresh and impactful.

In engaging with Yoga Nidra, individuals with fibromyalgia not only find a powerful tool for managing pain and enhancing sleep quality but also embark on a journey of self-discovery and healing. With its unique blend of relaxation, visualization, and intention, this practice offers more than temporary respite; it transforms how pain is perceived and experienced, inviting a deep connection with the inner self and a renewed sense of peace and wellbeing.

5.3 Loving-Kindness Meditation to Combat Loneliness

In the quiet spaces of the heart, where solitude often morphs into a sense of profound isolation, loving-kindness meditation (Metta Bhavana) emerges as a radiant beacon of compassion and connection. This ancient practice, rooted in the Buddhist tradition, extends an invitation to cultivate unconditional love and kindness towards oneself and others. At its core, loving-kindness meditation seeks to dissolve the barriers that separate us from the world, fostering a sense of deep, interconnected belonging that can be particularly therapeutic for those confronting the isolating experience of fibromyalgia.

The essence of loving-kindness meditation lies in its simplicity and profound potential for transformation. It begins with the self, for it is in nurturing self-compassion that we unlock the capacity to extend empathy and kindness to others. The practice involves the silent repetition of phrases imbued with warmth and goodwill, such as "May I be happy, may I be healthy, may I live with ease." These words, like seeds sown in the fertile soil of the mind, gradually take root, blossoming into a gentle acceptance and love of oneself, scars, and all.

Loving-kindness meditation starts with focusing on oneself and then extends outward to include loved ones, acquaintances, strangers, and even those with difficulties. This expansion is not merely an exercise in thought but a profound realignment of our relationship with the world. Each phrase, extended to another—"May you be happy, may you be healthy, may you live with ease"—becomes a bridge, connecting us through the shared desire for peace and wellbeing. This practice can transform perceived isolation into a deep connection by fostering empathy and understanding, reminding us of our shared humanity.

For individuals grappling with fibromyalgia, the feelings of loneliness and disconnection can be particularly acute. The physical limitations and persistent pain often create a chasm between the sufferer and the world around them, a gap that loving-kindness meditation seeks to bridge. The benefits for mental health are manifold; by cultivating a compassionate mindset, individuals report a significant decrease in feelings of isolation, depression, and anxiety. This shift is not merely psychological; the practice has been linked to physiological changes, including reduced stress levels and lower blood pressure, contributing to an overall sense of wellbeing.

Incorporating loving-kindness meditation into a regular meditation routine invites consistency and depth into the practice. It might begin with dedicating a few minutes at the start or end of each meditation session to loving-kindness, gradually allowing this focus on compassion to permeate the entire practice. For those navigating the challenges of fibromyalgia, integrating loving-kindness meditation can serve as a powerful counterbalance to the condition's isolating effects, fostering a sense of warmth and connectedness even on the most challenging days.

Furthermore, loving-kindness meditation can extend beyond the meditation cushion, with its principles woven into the fabric of everyday life. Simple acts, such as offering a smile to a stranger or extending patience and understanding to ourselves when we falter, embody the spirit of Metta. These acts, small in execution but vast in their ripple effects, reinforce the practice's teachings, embedding them into our interactions and internal monologue. This seamless integration of loving-kindness into daily life enhances our capacity for compassion and serves as a continual source of healing and connection.

In the silent communion with our deepest selves and the world around us, loving-kindness meditation offers a key to unlocking the doors of isolation imposed by fibromyalgia. It invites us into a realm where compassion is both sanctuary and bridge, where the warmth of our heart becomes the light that guides us back to a sense of belonging and peace. Through this practice, we learn that we are deeply connected to the vast web of life.

5.4 Zazen Practice: Sitting Meditation for Inner Peace

In the stillness that pervades the early morning air before the day's hustle begins, Zazen, a meditation practice steeped in the Zen Buddhism tradition, offers a sanctuary of calm and clarity. This practice, rooted in the principles of simplicity and observation, invites practitioners into a space of profound stillness and introspection. Originating from the serene monasteries of Japan, Zazen has transcended its ancient origins to become a beacon for those seeking solace and insight in the modern world. At its heart, Zazen is not merely a practice but a way of being, a pathway to experiencing life in its fullest, most vibrant form.

Zazen's essence lies in its unadorned simplicity, a direct encounter with the reality of the present moment. This practice eschews the complexity of rituals and mantras, focusing instead on the bare act of sitting and the subtle nuances of the mind in stillness. For individuals navigating the unpredictable waters of fibromyalgia, Zazen offers a stable anchor, a point of reference amid the fluctuating tides of pain and discomfort. It cultivates an environment where the physical challenges of fibromyalgia are met with a serene acceptance, transforming the relationship with pain from one of resistance to one of peaceful coexistence.

The foundation of Zazen's practice is proper posture and breath control, both simple in concept and profound in their impact. The posture, traditionally seated on a cushion with legs crossed in a lotus or half-lotus position, forms the physical framework for practice. This alignment, with the spine naturally straight and the hands resting gently on the lap, creates a stable yet relaxed structure conducive to deep meditation. The subtleties of this posture, from the slight tuck of the chin to the calm drop of the shoulders, are meticulously adjusted, ensuring that the body does not become a source of distraction but rather a vessel for deepening awareness.

Unlike practices that prescribe specific breathing patterns, breath control in Zazen emphasizes naturalness and ease. The breath can find its unforced and uncontrolled rhythm flowing freely in and out of the body. This attention to the breath, observed without alteration, becomes a powerful tool for anchoring the mind in the present, a gentle reminder to return whenever thoughts begin to wander. This focus on breathing, observed with gentle yet unwavering attention, cultivates a sense of inner calm, a softening of the mental and physical tensions that fibromyalgia so often exacerbates.

While straightforward, focusing the mind on Zazen unfolds as a subtle art, a delicate balancing act between attention and openness. For some, the practice involves the contemplation of koans, paradoxical questions, or statements that defy logical explanation, designed to transcend ordinary thinking, and provoke enlightenment. For others, the focus remains on the breath, observed with a keen and detached curiosity. This mental discipline, whether through koans or breath, trains the mind to dwell in a state of alert serenity, aware of thoughts and sensations as they arise but not trapped by them. This quality of mind, honed through regular Zazen practice, offers profound relief for those with fibromyalgia, providing a mental clarity that can illuminate the path through pain.

The principles of Zazen, grounded in mindfulness and presence, extend far beyond the cushion, weaving themselves into the fabric of daily life. This integration transforms ordinary moments into opportunities for meditation, inviting mindfulness that imbues even the most mundane tasks with a sense of purpose and presence. For individuals with fibromyalgia, this application of Zazen principles offers a way to navigate the day with increased awareness and equanimity, turning the challenges of chronic pain into moments of insight and growth. Whether in the deliberate savoring of a meal, the mindful completion of daily tasks, or the attentive listening in conversations, Zazen principles foster a way of living marked by a deep, abiding peace.

In the disciplined simplicity of Zazen, individuals find not only a method for managing the symptoms of fibromyalgia but also a profound way of engaging with the world. This practice, focusing on posture, breath, and mental focus, invites a journey inward to a place of stillness and insight where pain and discomfort are met with grace and acceptance. Through Zazen, the harsh landscape of fibromyalgia becomes a ground for cultivation, a place where the seeds of peace, clarity, and resilience are sown and nurtured. In this way, Zazen is more than a meditation practice; it is a pathway to a life lived with depth, purpose, and serenity, a testament to the enduring power of presence and mindfulness in the face of adversity.

5.5 Tapping into the Power of Chakra Meditation

The ancient system of chakras originates from Eastern spiritual traditions, mapping out the complex web of energy centers that govern our physical, emotional, and spiritual health. These swirling vortexes of energy, each associated with specific bodily regions and aspects of our wellbeing, serve as the foundation for chakra meditation. This practice seeks to align and balance these vital forces. For those grappling with the multifaceted symptoms of fibromyalgia, chakra meditation offers a unique lens through which to view and address their condition, promising pathways to relief that extend beyond the physical.

Navigating the intricacies of the chakra system illuminates the interconnectedness of our bodily systems and the energy that flows within. Starting from the root chakra at the base of the spine and ascending to the crown chakra at the top of the head, each energy center encapsulates specific facets of our being and potential blockages that can manifest as physical or emotional disturbances. The relevance of this system to fibromyalgia lies in its holistic approach to health, recognizing the ailment as a disruption not just of the body but of the energy that permeates it.

Embarking on chakra meditation for pain management involves:
- Focusing on engaging with each chakra.
- Identifying imbalances.
- Harnessing visualization and affirmations to restore equilibrium.

This process begins with grounding in the root chakra, envisioning a vibrant red energy that fosters a sense of safety and stability, counteracting the uncertainty and stress that fibromyalgia can induce. Progressing upward, attention shifts to the sacral chakra, whose orange glow represents creativity and emotional balance, and to the solar plexus chakra, where a bright yellow light signifies personal power and confidence—qualities often eroded by chronic illness.

Visualizations for chakra meditation draw upon the rich palette of colors associated with each energy center, imagining each chakra as a luminous, spinning wheel of light. For the heart chakra, radiant green energy encapsulates love and healing, directly addressing the emotional isolation that people living with fibromyalgia might experience. The throat chakra, bathed in soothing blue, empowers individuals to communicate their needs and experiences more openly, fostering a greater understanding and connection with those around them. Indigo light suffuses the third eye chakra, enhancing intuition and the ability to see beyond the pain. In contrast, the crown chakra glows with a violet light, connecting individuals to a sense of spiritual peace and purpose.

Affirmations complement these visualizations, with phrases tailored to each chakra's unique attributes. For instance, affirming "I am grounded and secure" reinforces the root chakra's energy, while "I express my truth freely" bolsters the throat chakra. These affirmations, repeated with conviction, act as seeds planted within the subconscious, gradually blooming into a profound internal shift that reflects in the physical realm. This synergy of visualization and affirmation, directed at the chakras most impacted by fibromyalgia, weaves a tapestry of healing that addresses the root causes of pain and imbalance.

Personal accounts from individuals who have integrated chakra meditation into their fibromyalgia management regimen attest to its transformative potential. One narrative describes a woman who noticed a significant reduction in her pain levels, improved sleep quality, and a newfound sense of emotional resilience after months of incorporating chakra meditation into her daily routine. Another recounts the journey of a man who found that focusing on his heart and solar plexus chakras brought him a deeper understanding of his condition and a greater capacity to cope with its challenges. These stories, each as unique as the individuals who share them, underscore the profound impact of chakra meditation, offering symptomatic relief and a more profound reconciliation with one's body and spirit.

Chakra meditation, with its rich history and integrated approach, stands as a beacon for those navigating the turbulent waters of fibromyalgia. It offers a method for managing pain and a deep spiritual practice that reconnects individuals to their innermost selves and the universal energy that binds us all. Through focused engagement with the chakra system, individuals find pathways to physical and emotional healing and greater harmony within themselves and the world around them.

5.6 Integrating Meditation with Daily Activities for Continuous Relief

The tapestry of daily life, woven with threads of routine and unexpected turns, holds within it the potential for a sanctuary. In this space, mindfulness transforms the mundane into moments of profound awareness and relief from the persistent whisper of fibromyalgia pain. This transformation requires not a retreat from the world but embracing it, with every action and interaction becoming a canvas for applying mindfulness techniques. In fully immersing oneself in the present, with every breath and movement, one finds a continuous stream of relief, a steady undercurrent of peace amidst the flux of chronic pain.

To infuse the day with mindfulness begins with setting intentions, a morning ritual that anchors the upcoming activities in a conscious awareness. Before the sun casts its first light, a quiet reflection on the day's aspirations lays the groundwork for a mindful approach to routine tasks and pain management. This intention might be as simple as focusing on the breath during daily commutes or as profound as embodying compassion in every interaction. The significance of this practice lies not in the grandeur of the intention but in its capacity to direct the mind and serve as a compass guiding one's actions and reactions through the lens of mindfulness.

Reminders, strategically placed within the day's landscape, act as buoys, gently steering one back to the present whenever the mind drifts into the turbulent waters of pain or stress. These can take myriad forms, from alarms on a digital device that prompt a minute of deep breathing to tactile cues like wearing a specific piece of jewelry that, upon touch, serves as a call to return to mindfulness. Opening a door can become a reminder, a pause in which one takes a deep breath and re-center. These subtle nudges maintain the continuity of mindfulness throughout the day, weaving a thread of awareness that connects each moment to the next.

Integrating mindfulness into daily activities transforms even the most ordinary tasks into meditation practices. Washing dishes, the hands immersed in warm, soapy water becomes an exercise in sensory awareness, with attention paid to the texture of the bubbles, the sound of water splashing, and the rhythm of the breath. Eating, too, offers a rich opportunity for mindfulness, with each bite savored, each flavor and texture noted with appreciation. This approach, where activities become conduits for mindfulness, not only enriches the experience of the present but also creates a buffer against the intrusion of pain, offering relief in the gentle focus on the now.

A reflective practice offers insights into how integrating meditation into daily life impacts fibromyalgia symptoms and overall wellbeing.

This might involve a nightly journaling exercise in which you record reflections on the day's moments of mindfulness, the challenges you faced, and the relief you experienced. Through this lens, the fluctuations in pain levels, the moments of peace amidst discomfort, and the overall trajectory of one's wellbeing come into sharp relief. This practice highlights the tangible benefits of mindfulness and reinforces the commitment to this approach, affirming its value in the continuous management of fibromyalgia.

As this chapter finds its close, the threads of mindfulness woven throughout the day emerge not as isolated practices but as a cohesive tapestry of awareness and relief. The integration of meditation into daily activities, from the setting of intentions to the use of reminders, the mindful execution of tasks, and the reflective evaluation of progress, creates a foundation for continuous relief from fibromyalgia pain. This approach, rooted in the present and rich in simplicity, offers a method for managing symptoms and a way of living intensely, fully aware, and appreciative of each moment. As we transition from the exploration of mindfulness in the day-to-day to the broader landscape of holistic health, this foundation of mindfulness serves as a cornerstone, a steady base upon which to build a comprehensive strategy for wellbeing that addresses the body, mind, and spirit.

Chapter 6 Lifestyle Modifications for Managing Fibromyalgia

In the clamor of day-to-day existence, sleep often falls to the wayside, relegated to an afterthought amid the rush of obligations and the pervasive hum of technology. Yet, for those entwined in the persistent embrace of fibromyalgia, sleep transforms from a mere nightly ritual into a crucible of rest and recovery. The delicate balance between refreshing slumber and the tendrils of pain and fatigue becomes a pivotal arena in the quest for wellbeing. This chapter narrows to the intricate dance between sleep and fibromyalgia, unraveling how one influences the other and laying out strategies to enhance the quality of rest.

6.1 The Impact of Sleep on Fibromyalgia and How to Improve It

The connection between sleep and pain

The relationship between sleep and fibromyalgia is a complex ballet, where disruption in one invariably influences the other. Poor sleep exacerbates the symptoms of fibromyalgia, heightening pain sensitivity and fogging the mind, while the relentless grip of fibromyalgia pain makes the prospect

A peaceful night's slumber seems like a distant dream. This cycle, a feedback loop of discomfort and restlessness, underscores the necessity of addressing sleep quality as a cornerstone of fibromyalgia management. Studies have illuminated that enhancing sleep quality can significantly reduce pain, highlighting the need for targeted sleep interventions.

Sleep hygiene practices

Creating a sanctuary of sleep involves more than just a comfortable mattress or a darkened room. It is about fostering an environment and a routine conducive to deep, restorative rest. Establishing a consistent sleep schedule is the first step, aligning the body's internal clock with a regular pattern of rest and wakefulness. Dimming lights and disconnecting from screens an hour before bedtime reduces blue light exposure, signaling the brain that it is time to wind down. Dimming lights and disconnecting from screens an hour before bedtime decreases the intrusion of blue light, signaling to the brain that it is time to wind down. The bedroom, reserved for sleep and intimacy alone, becomes a cue for relaxation, free from the distractions of work or entertainment. Comfort is critical in this space, so adjust the room temperature, bedding, and sleepwear to your preferences to ensure the physical conditions are primed for sleep.

Relaxation techniques for better sleep

On the cusp of sleep, when the mind teeters between wakefulness and rest, relaxation techniques can serve as a bridge to the land of dreams. Guided imagery, where one visualizes a serene setting or a tranquil experience, acts as a mental escape from the tight grip of pain and anxiety. Through its systematic tensing and relaxing of muscle groups, progressive muscle relaxation releases the day's accumulated tension, smoothing the transition into sleep. Deep breathing exercises, with their rhythmic inhale and exhale, become a lullaby, lulling the body into a state of relaxation. Incorporating these practices into the pre-sleep routine can significantly improve the ease of falling asleep and the depth of rest.

When to seek professional help

There are moments when the strategies and routines designed to foster sleep fall short, and the specter of insomnia looms large. Recognizing the signs that professional intervention may be required is crucial. If sleep disturbances persist despite adherence to sleep hygiene practices, or if waking up feeling unrefreshed becomes the norm rather than the exception, it may be time to consult a healthcare provider. Sleep disorders such as sleep apnea, restless legs syndrome, or periodic limb movement disorder, which are more common among those with fibromyalgia, require specialized treatment. A sleep specialist can offer tailored advice, conduct sleep studies, and prescribe interventions that address the barriers to restorative sleep faced by individuals with fibromyalgia.

Textual Element: Sleep Hygiene Checklist

- **Establish a consistent sleep schedule:** Go to bed and wake up simultaneously every day, even on weekends.

- **Create a bedtime ritual**: Before bed, engage in relaxing activities such as reading, taking a warm bath, or practicing relaxation techniques.
- **Optimize your sleep environment**: Ensure your bedroom is dark, quiet, and calm. Consider using blackout curtains, earplugs, or a white noise machine if necessary.
- **Limit exposure to screens**: Avoid using electronic devices at least an hour before bedtime to reduce blue light exposure.
- **Be mindful of food and drink**: Avoid heavy meals, caffeine, and alcohol close to bedtime.
- **Reserve the bed for sleep and intimacy**: Avoid working, eating, or watching TV in bed to strengthen the association between your bed and sleep.

Incorporating these practices and being attuned to the body's signals allows for a proactive and responsive approach to sleep, weaving a tapestry of night-time habits that support the journey towards improved wellbeing for those with fibromyalgia.

6.2 Gentle Physical Exercises Tailored for Senior Women

In the quiet tapestry of managing fibromyalgia, the thread of physical activity weaves a pattern of nuanced relief and empowerment. For senior women, this thread holds particular significance, as the challenges of fibromyalgia intertwine with the natural considerations of aging. The dance of exercise and fibromyalgia is intricate, requiring a balance between movement and rest, between pushing the boundaries and heeding the body's whispers of limitation.

Physical activity, often viewed through the lens of vigor and intensity, finds a gentle counterpart in fibromyalgia management. Here, the benefits of exercise unfurl in the subtle alleviation of symptoms, in the increased flexibility of joints encased in stiffness, and in the quiet strengthening of muscles too long held captive by pain. This movement, far from the robust exertions of youth, embraces a softer approach that nurtures the body while coaxing it towards wellness.

For senior women navigating the waters of fibromyalgia, low-impact exercises emerge as beacons of hope. With its rhythmic, soothing cadence, activities such as walking offer a form of cardiovascular exercise that respects the body's need for gentleness. Water aerobics, performed in the supportive embrace of water, reduces the strain on painful joints, allowing for freedom of movement that dry land seldom affords. With its deliberate, flowing motions, Tai Chi enhances physical balance and instills a sense of inner calm. This meditative quality addresses the mind-body connection central to fibromyalgia management. Yoga is adapted to accommodate the limitations fibromyalgia imposes, stretches, and strengthens the body while fostering an environment of deep breathing and relaxation.

Incorporating these activities into the fabric of daily life requires a thoughtful, gradual approach. It begins with acknowledging current physical capabilities and setting aside the urge to compare today's abilities with those of the past. From this starting point, small increments of activity are introduced, a short walk in the early morning when the world is still, and the body is most receptive to movement. This walk, initially brief, lengthens over time as the body adapts, building stamina and resilience. Similarly, sessions of water aerobics or Tai Chi begin with once-weekly attendance, slowly increasing in frequency as the benefits become apparent and the body's capacity for exercise grows.

Listening to the body is the guiding principle in this gradual integration of exercise. It is a dialogue, a continuous conversation in which the body speaks in sensations of comfort and discomfort, and the mind listens with attentiveness and respect. On days when pain flares, this listening may dictate a lighter routine, gentle stretching, or a restful pause from activity altogether. On days when the body hums with a readiness for movement, slightly more ambitious exercises might be embraced. This attunement prevents overexertion, a critical consideration, as pushing beyond the body's limits can exacerbate fibromyalgia symptoms rather than alleviate them.

Pain induced by exercise, a concern for many with fibromyalgia, is addressed not through avoidance but through strategic management. Cooling down after physical activity, with stretches that gently coax the muscles back into a state of rest, reduces the likelihood of post-exercise discomfort. Applying heat to sore areas, through warm baths or heating pads, offers solace to muscles tender from the exertion. Moreover, the scheduling of exercise, timed to coincide with natural peaks in energy and to avoid the hours when pain typically intensifies, further mitigates the risk of exercise-induced pain.

A landscape of potential unfolds in the realm of gentle physical exercises tailored for senior women with fibromyalgia. It is a domain where movement whispers secrets of strength and resilience to bodies wearied by pain, where every step, stretch, and breath of effort brings physical benefits and a reclamation of agency over one's wellbeing. This approach to exercise, characterized by its gentleness and adaptability, becomes not just a method of managing fibromyalgia symptoms but a celebration of what the body can still achieve, a testament to the enduring spirit of those who move through the world with grace despite the challenges they face.

6.3 The Role of Hydration and Nutrition in Pain Management

Within the labyrinth of fibromyalgia management, the alchemy of hydration and nutrition emerges as a pivotal element, wielding the power to modulate the intensity of symptoms with a subtlety that belies its profound impact. The intricate dance between what we consume and the echoes of discomfort that fibromyalgia casts across the body's landscape necessitates a careful curation of dietary choices, transforming the act of eating and drinking into a deliberate strategy for symptom relief.

Nutritional Considerations for Fibromyalgia

The dialogue between fibromyalgia symptoms and the spectrum of foods and nutrients available to us is nuanced, characterized by both the potential to soothe and the capability to inflame. Foods act as kindling to the smoldering flames of fibromyalgia pain, with processed sugars, refined carbohydrates, and saturated fats playing leading roles in this exacerbation. Conversely, adopting a diet rich in omega-3 fatty acids found abundantly in fish like salmon and flaxseeds introduces a counter-narrative where inflammation is quelled, and pain is subdued. Antioxidant-rich fruits and vegetables, in their vibrant array of colors and nutrients, contribute to this symphony of relief, their bioactive compounds acting as scavengers of the free radicals implicated in the pain pathways of fibromyalgia. Including whole grains and lean proteins rounds out this dietary strategy, providing sustained energy and supporting muscle health; both are critical for navigating the energy troughs and physical discomforts characteristic of fibromyalgia.

Hydration and Its Effects on Pain

The act of hydration, mundane in its simplicity, holds the key to alleviating the multifaceted symptoms of fibromyalgia. Water, the most unassuming of beverages, can lubricate joints, flush toxins, and ensure the optimal functioning of cells, including those responsible for transmitting pain signals. Dehydration, often an overlooked companion of daily life, subtly tightens its grip on the body, exacerbating muscle soreness and amplifying pain perception. Therefore, maintaining adequate hydration becomes not just a recommendation but a necessity, with the intake of fluids tailored to individual needs and activity levels. Incorporating herbal teas adds complexity to this hydration strategy, with specific blends offering additional benefits such as muscle relaxation and improved digestion, further supporting the body's resilience against the onslaught of fibromyalgia symptoms.

Creating a Balanced Diet

The blueprint for a diet that supports the management of fibromyalgia symptoms emphasizes balance and variety, crafting a nutritional tapestry that nourishes the body while simultaneously countering inflammation and pain. This dietary approach begins with abundant fruits and vegetables, their natural phytochemicals acting as allies in the battle against oxidative stress and inflammation. With their rich fiber content, whole grains play a dual role, contributing to digestive health and providing a steady energy source, vital for combating fatigue that often shadows fibromyalgia. Lean proteins, whether from plant or animal sources, supply the building blocks for muscle repair and maintenance, a critical consideration for bodies beleaguered by pain. Healthy fats, those rich in omega-3 fatty acids, weave through this dietary fabric, offering anti-inflammatory benefits and supporting brain health. The careful calibration of meal timing and portion sizes further refines this approach, ensuring that the body receives a steady stream of nutrients without the strain of digesting large, infrequent meals.

Supplements and Fibromyalgia

In the realm of fibromyalgia management, dietary supplements stand at the crossroads of controversy and hope, offering the promise of symptom relief against a backdrop of scientific scrutiny. The judicious use of supplements, informed by both research and individual health profiles, can address specific nutritional deficiencies that may exacerbate fibromyalgia symptoms. Magnesium, known for its role in muscle relaxation and nerve function, emerges as a candidate for supplementation, particularly in individuals whose dietary intake falls short of the recommended levels. Similarly, vitamin D, often lacking due to limited sun exposure and dietary sources, holds the potential to modulate pain perception and improve overall wellbeing. Supplementing omega-3 fatty acids for those whose diets lack sufficient fatty fish or plant-based sources offers another avenue for reducing inflammation and pain. It is imperative, however, that the introduction of any supplement into one's regimen is preceded by a thorough consultation with a healthcare provider, ensuring that the benefits outweigh the risks and that the chosen supplements harmonize with any existing treatments.

A narrative of empowerment and intentionality unfolds in navigating the complexities of hydration and nutrition within the context of fibromyalgia management. This journey through food, fluids, and supplements is not a quest for a panacea but a pursuit of balance, a series of choices that collectively wield the power to modulate symptoms and enhance the quality of life. The alchemy of combining the proper nutrients with adequate hydration, tailored to the unique needs of everyone, crafts a foundation upon which the management of fibromyalgia symptoms rests, transforming the act of nourishment into a deliberate strategy for wellbeing.

6.4 Environmental Adjustments for Better Living with Fibromyalgia

Amidst the tapestry of managing fibromyalgia, the home environment and daily living practices play a pivotal role, often overlooked, in moderating the ebb and flow of symptoms. The spaces we inhabit and the clothes we drape over our bodies carry an unspoken power, profoundly influencing our comfort and wellbeing. Crafting a living space that acknowledges and accommodates the unique sensitivities associated with fibromyalgia not only mitigates the discomfort but also fosters a sanctuary of relief and tranquility.

Creating a Fibro-Friendly Home

Transforming a home into a fibro-friendly haven begins with an awareness of the sensory triggers that can precipitate flare-ups. Bright lights and loud sounds, for instance, not only assault the senses but can also heighten pain perception. Dimmer switches install a measure of control over lighting intensity, allowing for the softening of harsh glares that can fatigue the eyes and exacerbate headaches. Similarly, the strategic placement of rugs and curtains can dampen noise, creating pockets of serenity in a world that often throws with too much intensity. Furniture selection, too, holds the key to comfort; supportive seating and mattresses tailored to alleviate pressure points can transform hours of potential discomfort into moments of reprieve.

Ergonomic Considerations

The principle of ergonomics, focused on optimizing human wellbeing and overall system performance, finds its relevance magnified within the context of fibromyalgia. Daily tasks can become Herculean trials when pain and fatigue loom large. Ergonomic tools designed to minimize strain offer a bridge across these trials. Adjustable chairs and desks that cater to a natural posture, keyboard and mouse setups that reduce wrist strain, and kitchen utensils with easy-to-grip handles all contribute to a living environment that supports rather than challenges. These adjustments, subtle yet impactful, weave a thread of ease through the fabric of daily living, reducing the physical stressors that can trigger fibromyalgia symptoms.

Temperature and Clothing

Sensitivity to temperature fluctuations, an everyday companion to fibromyalgia, calls for an adaptive approach to home environment and personal attire. The layering of clothing, embracing materials that breathe and insulate according to the body's shifting needs, offers a strategy to navigate the discomfort of sudden temperature changes. Similarly, the home becomes a responsive habitat, with fans, heaters, and adjustable thermostats providing a means to address discomfort quickly. In this dance with temperature, materials come to the fore; natural fibers that wick away moisture and maintain breathability stand out as allies, clothing the body in comfort that adjusts with the thermometer's whims.

Accessibility and Mobility Aids

The acknowledgment of mobility as a variable rather than a constant underscores the necessity for accessibility adjustments within the home. Rugs that slip, bathtubs that present insurmountable barriers, and cabinets that stretch beyond reach pose unnecessary challenges. Addressing these through non-slip mats, walk-in showers with grab bars, and reorganized living spaces that place frequently used items within easy reach respects the body's fluctuating capabilities. Mobility aids, from canes that provide stability to wheelchairs that offer freedom of movement, should not be viewed as concessions to fibromyalgia but as tools of empowerment, extensions of the self that navigates the world gracefully. These aids and adjustments do not signify a relinquishing of independence but a reclaiming of autonomy, a reconfiguration of the environment to support rather than constrain.

Through these environmental and lifestyle adjustments, the home transitions from a mere backdrop to an active participant in managing fibromyalgia. Each modification, each choice in attire or furniture, becomes a statement of resilience, a declaration that living with fibromyalgia is not merely about enduring but about thriving within the spaces we call our own. This approach to crafting a fibro-friendly living environment does not seek to eliminate the challenges of fibromyalgia but to mitigate its impact, creating a buffer of comfort and convenience against the condition's unpredictability. In this way, the home becomes not just a place of refuge but a space of empowerment, a setting where the narrative of fibromyalgia is one of adaptation and strength, woven into the very fabric of daily life.

6.5 The Power of a Strong Support System

In the tapestry of managing fibromyalgia, threads of solitude often weave through the fabric of daily life, creating a pattern of isolation that can weigh heavily on the spirit. Yet, amidst this solitude, a robust support system emerges as a beacon of light, illuminating pathways to resilience and wellbeing. Cultivating this network—comprising family, friends, healthcare providers, and caregivers—transforms the solitary journey into a shared voyage marked by empathy, understanding, and collective strength.

Building a Support Network

The architecture of a supportive network requires intentionality, a deliberate effort to draw together individuals whose presence nurtures and sustains. This diverse network offers a multifaceted support structure, with each member contributing their unique perspective, experience, and strength. With their intimate knowledge of the individual's history and personality, family and friends provide emotional comfort and a sense of belonging. Healthcare providers, armed with their expertise, guide the journey with clinical advice, treatment options, and ongoing care. Together, these relationships form the pillars of a support system that upholds the individual through the ebbs and flows of managing fibromyalgia.

Communicating Needs

The foundation of this support system rests on clear, open communication—a sharing of needs, limitations, and aspirations that invites understanding and empathy. Articulating the intricacies of fibromyalgia to those unfamiliar with its challenges requires patience and clarity, an education that bridges gaps in knowledge. This communication extends to expressing when help is needed, whether in managing daily tasks, navigating healthcare decisions, or simply seeking solace in moments of distress. Voicing these needs without fear of judgment or burden deepens the connection with one's support network, ensuring that assistance aligns with the individual's wishes and requirements.

Finding Community

Beyond the immediate circle of personal contacts, the community search connects individuals with fibromyalgia to a broader network of peers navigating similar challenges. Support groups, whether found in local community centers or the digital realms of online forums and social media, offer spaces of shared experience and collective wisdom. Bound by everyday struggles and victories, these communities provide a platform for exchange— of coping strategies, treatment experiences, and emotional support. Sharing one's story and hearing those of others validates individual experiences, mitigating feelings of isolation and fostering a sense of camaraderie and mutual support.

The Role of Caregivers

Within the constellation of support, caregivers occupy a pivotal role, their presence a constant source of assistance, encouragement, and care. These individuals, whether family members, friends, or professionals, navigate the complexities of fibromyalgia alongside those they support, often adjusting their own lives to accommodate the needs of their loved ones. The role of caregivers extends beyond physical assistance; it encompasses emotional support, advocacy in healthcare settings, and collaboration in lifestyle modifications. Recognizing and appreciating caregivers' efforts while respecting their needs and boundaries strengthens this vital relationship, ensuring that it remains sustainable and mutually beneficial.

In fibromyalgia management, the power of a robust support system cannot be overstated. This network, woven from the threads of shared experiences, empathy, and care, offers a foundation of strength upon which individuals can build a life of resilience and wellbeing. Through clear communication, fostering community, and nurturing caregiver relationships, the journey through fibromyalgia becomes a shared voyage, marked not by solitude but by the collective endeavor to thrive amidst the challenges.

6.6 Managing Stress Through Time Management and Prioritization

Within the intricate dance of living with fibromyalgia, stress acts as both a catalyst and an amplifier of the condition's myriad symptoms. The body, trapped in a constant state of alert, finds little respite from the relentless cycle of discomfort and fatigue, rendering stress a psychological burden and a physical albatross. Therefore, the criticality of mitigating stress cannot be overstated; it demands a strategic approach that intertwines the threads of time management and prioritization into a cohesive fabric of wellbeing. When applied to the realities of fibromyalgia, the ethos of effective time management transcends the conventional boundaries of productivity. It becomes a deliberate act of self-preservation, a means to delineate the finite reserves of energy from the infinite demands of daily life. Practical strategies begin with the meticulous planning of tasks, employing tools such as calendars and to-do lists not as mere organizational aids but as instruments of empowerment. This planning entails the enumeration of tasks and an honest assessment of their urgency and importance, a distinction that allows for the reasonable allocation of one's energy.

Prioritization emerges as a companion to time management, a discerning eye that identifies tasks that align with personal values and goals while relegating less consequential activities to the periphery. This exercise in discernment, however, demands flexibility, an acknowledgment that the unpredictable nature of fibromyalgia may necessitate adjustments to the best-laid plans. The art of saying no, an often-overlooked facet of prioritization, becomes a powerful tool in this context, enabling individuals to safeguard their time and energy against commitments that detract from their wellbeing.

Integrating relaxation and self-care into one's daily schedule is a non-negotiable pillar of managing stress. These activities, far from indulgent, act as critical counterbalances to the rigors of fibromyalgia, restoring a sense of calm and equilibrium to a body often in turmoil. Relaxation techniques, from deep breathing exercises to guided meditations, offer accessible pathways to tranquility, their regular practice weaving a protective barrier against the encroachment of stress. Self-care, in its myriad forms, from engaging in hobbies to connecting with loved ones, replenishes the spirit, fortifying the individual against the psychological and physical onslaught of fibromyalgia.

The encapsulation of stress management within the context of fibromyalgia draws a map through the terrain of time management and prioritization, charting a course toward reduced symptom severity and enhanced quality of life. This journey, marked by deliberate planning, discerning prioritization, and the integration of relaxation, underscores the possibility of navigating fibromyalgia with grace and resilience. It highlights the power inherent in reclaiming control over one's time and energy, transforming the narrative of living with fibromyalgia from endurance to empowerment.

In weaving the principles of time management and prioritization into the fabric of daily life, individuals with fibromyalgia forge a shield against stress. This bulwark guards not just against the worsening of symptoms but against the erosion of quality of life. This approach, rooted in strategy and self-compassion, offers not a cure but a means to live more fully and navigate the complexities of fibromyalgia with a sense of agency and purpose. As we turn the page, we carry forward the lessons of mindfulness and intentionality, embarking on a continued exploration of strategies that support living well with fibromyalgia.

Chapter 7 Addressing Common Challenges and Objections

In the realm of fibromyalgia management, a sentiment often emerges from the depths of frustration and fatigue: "I've tried everything." More than a mere expression of Despair, this statement encapsulates the cyclical battle between hope and disillusionment that defines the condition. It reflects the countless attempts to find solace in treatments that promise relief, only to be met with the stubborn persistence of pain. However, beneath this veneer of defeat lies an opportunity for transformation, a reorientation towards a path marked not by the elusive promise of a cure but by the tangible reality of effective management and enhanced quality of life.

7.1 "I've Tried Everything": Overcoming Despair

Recognizing the Cycle of Despair
The cyclical nature of Despair in fibromyalgia can often feel akin to Sisyphus's eternal struggle, pushing a boulder up a hill only to roll down each time it nears the summit. This analogy, while ancient, resonates with the modern experience of fibromyalgia—each failed treatment attempt adds weight to the burden of pain. Recognizing this cycle is the first step towards breaking it, acknowledging that both setbacks and advances punctuate the journey through fibromyalgia. It is a process of learning and adaptation, where each attempt, regardless of its outcome, contributes to a deeper understanding of one's condition.

Reframing the Journey
Reframing the journey through fibromyalgia involves shifting focus from the pursuit of a cure to the pursuit of management strategies that enhance quality of life. This perspective acknowledges fibromyalgia as a part of one's life but not the entirety of it. It is about finding value in the small victories—moments of relief, however fleeting, that collectively weave a tapestry of a life of purpose and joy. This reframing is not resignation but a pragmatic acknowledgment of the condition's complexity, fostering resilience and a sense of agency.

Exploring Underutilized Options
The medical landscape is ever evolving, with new treatments and lifestyle adjustments emerging that may offer relief. For instance, integrating complementary therapies such as acupuncture or myofascial release therapy into one's treatment plan can target pain from different angles. Similarly, advancements in nutritional science suggest the role of certain

diets in modulating the inflammatory processes associated with fibromyalgia. Exploring these underutilized options requires an open dialogue with healthcare providers, a willingness to experiment, and an understanding that what works is highly individualized.

The Power of Incremental Changes

The cumulative effect of small, sustainable changes often goes unnoticed in the quest for immediate relief. Yet, these incremental adjustments—a gentle stretching routine incorporated into the morning, a mindfulness practice before bed, and the gradual reconfiguration of dietary habits—build the foundation for long-term management. This approach mirrors the concept of kaizen, a philosophy of continuous improvement where small, consistent actions leads to significant changes over time. Applying this principle to fibromyalgia management empowers individuals to take active steps toward relief, one minor change at a time.

Textual Element: Lifestyle Adjustment Checklist

- **Morning Routine**: Incorporate a 10-minute gentle stretching or yoga session to ease morning stiffness.
- **Nutritional Tweaks**: Gradually increase intake of anti-inflammatory foods such as leafy greens, nuts, and fatty fish while reducing processed foods.
- **Mindfulness Practice**: Dedicate 5 minutes before bed to a mindfulness or visualization exercise to promote relaxation and improve sleep quality.
- **Activity Journal**: Keep a daily log of activities, noting how each affects fibromyalgia symptoms, to identify patterns and potential triggers.
- **Hydration Reminder**: Set reminders to drink water throughout the day, aiming for at least eight glasses to aid in toxin removal and muscle function.

This checklist, while simple, encapsulates the essence of incremental change—small actions that, when consistently applied, can shift the trajectory of fibromyalgia management from Despair to empowerment. It is a tangible expression of the adage that the journey of a thousand miles begins with a single step, a reminder that in the realm of fibromyalgia, progress is measured not by the disappearance of symptoms but by the enhancement of life's quality amidst their presence.

7.2 Meditation Misconceptions: "It's Not for Me"

Debunking Meditation Myths

In the quiet spaces between our constant thoughts and the relentless pace of life, meditation offers a sanctuary of calm—a respite from the tumult of daily existence and, for those with fibromyalgia, the constant echo of pain. Yet, with its promise of peace and mindfulness, this ancient practice often encounters resistance, shrouded as it is in misconceptions and myths. The first is the belief that meditation requires an empty mind, a state of thoughtless serenity that, to many, seems unattainable amidst the chatter of the internal dialogue. However, the essence of meditation lies not in eradicating thoughts but in observing them without attachment, letting them drift by like leaves on a stream, acknowledging their presence but not holding on to them.

Another pervasive myth is the notion that meditation demands uncomfortable physical postures; hours spent in lotus position with legs entwined in configurations that challenge even the flexible. This image dissuades many, particularly those for whom fibromyalgia renders such positions not just uncomfortable but unfeasible. Yet, meditation, in its inclusivity, asks not for contortion but for comfort, allowing for a multitude of postures that can accommodate any level of flexibility. Sitting on a chair with feet planted firmly on the ground, lying down, or even strolling in a quiet space—all these are valid doors to the state of mindfulness that meditation seeks to cultivate.

Showcasing Variety in Meditation

The landscape of meditation is vast and varied, a testament to the myriad ways humans have sought inner peace and connection through the ages. Beyond the widely recognized practice of mindfulness meditation, with its focus on breath and present-moment awareness, lies a rich tapestry of techniques, each with its unique approach to fostering tranquility and insight. For instance, loving-kindness meditation extends compassion towards oneself and others, a practice particularly poignant for those grappling with the isolation and frustration that fibromyalgia often brings. Visualization meditation invites practitioners to journey inward to serene landscapes or healing processes, offering distraction and solace from physical discomfort.

Transcendental Meditation, with its use of mantras, offers a different path of repetition and focus that can lead to deep relaxation and stress reduction. Similarly, Zen meditation, or Zazen, emphasizes simplicity and observation, a practice of just sitting and being that can be profoundly grounding for those adrift in the sea of chronic pain. Each of these practices, with its unique focus and technique, underscores the accessibility of meditation, revealing it as a practice not confined by rigid rules but open to interpretation and adaptation.

Personal Stories of Transformation

Amid meditation's skepticism, personal narratives are powerful testaments to their transformative potential. Take, for example, the story of Maria, a woman in her late sixties grappling with fibromyalgia's relentless grip. For Maria, meditation was a foreign concept, associated more with ascetics and monastics than practical pain management. Yet, driven by a desire for relief and a sense of desperation, she embarked on a journey through mindfulness, initially struggling with her racing thoughts and the discomfort of sitting still. Over time, however, she noticed a shift—a gradual easing of her pain and an increased capacity to manage flare-ups with a calmness that was previously foreign to her.

Then there's John, a retired teacher whose diagnosis of fibromyalgia threatened to overshadow his golden years. John found solace in loving-kindness meditation, which alleviated his sense of isolation and infused his daily interactions with warmth and patience that transformed his relationships. These stories, and countless others like them, illuminate the diverse pathways through which meditation can impact lives, offering symptomatic relief and a profound reconnection with the self and the world.

Guidance for Beginners

For those standing at the threshold of this practice, uncertain of how to proceed, the initiation into meditation need not be daunting. Beginning with just a few minutes a day, finding a quiet space where interruptions are few, and adopting a comfortable posture, one can start the journey towards mindfulness. Guided meditations, available through apps or online platforms, can provide direction, offering a gentle introduction to the practice. It is essential, too, to approach meditation with patience and self-compassion, understanding that distraction and wandering thoughts are not failures but part of the process. As familiarity with the practice grows, so does the ability to linger longer in the spaces between thoughts, finding peace in those moments that transcend the physical confines of pain.

This exploration of meditation, with its debunking of myths, introduction to the variety of practices, sharing of personal stories, and guidance for beginners, illuminates a path forward for those with fibromyalgia—a path marked not by the elusive goal of an empty mind but by the tangible, accessible practice of presence and mindfulness.

7.3 Simplifying CBT: It is Easier Than You Think

Demystifying CBT

Cognitive Behavioral Therapy, often shrouded in the misconception of being an intricate, therapist-only domain, operates on the foundational principle that our thoughts, feelings, and behaviors are intricately linked, influencing, and being influenced by one another. At its heart, CBT is a dialogue—a conversation with oneself aimed at identifying and adjusting the patterns of thinking that contribute to the distressing tapestry of fibromyalgia symptoms. This self-dialogue, far from the daunting task, is a skill that can be honed, transforming how pain is perceived and managed. The essence of CBT lies in its simplicity and adaptability, making it an accessible tool for those beyond the therapist's office, a means to gently rewire the neural pathways carved by chronic pain.

Self-administered CBT Techniques

The journey into self-administered CBT begins with thought recording—a simple yet profound technique of noting down thoughts as they arise, particularly those that flutter through the mind in moments of pain or discomfort. This recording, akin to laying the puzzle pieces on a table, offers a tangible view of the mental landscape, revealing patterns and recurrent themes in one's thought processes. The next step, though challenging, involves a gentle interrogation of these recorded thoughts, questioning their validity and exploring the evidence that supports or contradicts them. Though initially unsettling, this process gradually fosters a shift towards more balanced, less distressing patterns of thinking.

For instance, the thought "I will never find relief from this pain" can be challenged with evidence of past moments of comfort, however brief, or instances when adjustments in treatment or lifestyle brought measurable improvements in symptoms. This technique of challenging and reframing thoughts is not an attempt to dismiss the reality of fibromyalgia but a strategy to reduce the additional layer of suffering that arises from catastrophizing and pessimistic thinking. Incorporating behavioral experiments, another facet of self-administered CBT invites individuals to test the beliefs that fuel their distress. By engaging in activities previously avoided due to fear of exacerbating pain and observing the outcomes, a more nuanced understanding of one's capabilities and limits emerges, often revealing that the boundaries of possibility are wider than initially perceived.

Accessing CBT Resources

The digital age has ushered in a wealth of resources, making the principles and practices of CBT more accessible than ever. Books penned by professionals in the field offer deep dives into the theory behind CBT and provide step-by-step guides for applying its techniques. Online courses, ranging from introductory overviews to more in-depth explorations, cater to varying levels of familiarity with CBT, allowing for self-paced learning. Apps designed to facilitate CBT practices, from thought recording to mood tracking, offer a portable means of integrating CBT into daily life, turning spare moments into opportunities for reflection and growth. These resources, by demystifying CBT and breaking down its components into digestible, actionable steps, empower individuals to take an active role in managing their fibromyalgia.

Success with CBT

The narrative of fibromyalgia, often marked by chapters of frustration and pain, finds moments of hope in the success stories of those who have woven CBT into their management strategy. Consider the tale of a person who, after years of battling with the pervasive fog of fibromyalgia, discovered in CBT a clarity that pierced through the haze. Through diligent application of thought recording and challenging, this individual gradually shifted from a stance of helplessness to one of empowerment, finding in the nuances of their thought patterns the keys to unlocking a more manageable existence with fibromyalgia. Another recounts the liberation found in behavioral experiments, where the gradual re-engagement with physical activities, once abandoned in fear, led to a rekindling of joy and a sense of accomplishment that fibromyalgia had long eclipsed.

These stories, each unique in their contours, share a common thread—the transformative impact of CBT on the experience of fibromyalgia. They serve as testaments to the potential that lies in the deliberate examination and adjustment of our thoughts and behaviors, a reminder that within the realm of chronic pain, there exists the possibility for change, for a life defined not by the limitations of fibromyalgia but by the resilience and adaptability of the human spirit. Through CBT, individuals gain not just a strategy for coping with symptoms but also a new perspective that allows them to view the challenges of fibromyalgia with renewed hope and agency.

7.4 Beyond Medication: Exploring Nonpharmacological Treatments

In the vast landscape of fibromyalgia management, a realm extends far beyond the boundaries of conventional medication. This domain, rich with the potential for pain relief and symptom management, embraces the holistic ethos of treating the individual as a whole—mind, body, and spirit. Within this approach, an array of nonpharmacological treatments emerges, each with its unique contribution to the tapestry of care for those living with fibromyalgia. Physical therapy, acupuncture, and nutritional adjustments stand as pillars within this realm, offering avenues for relief that complement the pharmacological strategies often at the forefront of fibromyalgia treatment.

Physical therapy, with its foundation in the science of movement, offers a tailored approach to managing fibromyalgia symptoms. Through targeted exercises, individuals regain strength, flexibility, and endurance, countering the muscle stiffness and weakness that fibromyalgia often engenders. A skilled physical therapist's therapeutic hands also guide patients through pain management techniques, including heat and cold therapy, electrical stimulation, and myofascial release. These modalities, grounded in evidence of their efficacy, provide symptomatic relief and a pathway to improved functionality and quality of life. The deliberate, focused movements and therapies employed in physical therapy sessions act as a balm to the overstimulated nervous system, dialing down the volume of pain signals and fostering a sense of bodily autonomy that fibromyalgia often erodes.

Acupuncture, a practice with roots in ancient Chinese medicine, introduces a different dimension to fibromyalgia management. This technique involves the insertion of fine needles into specific points on the body, a process that, according to traditional beliefs, restores the balance of energy, or qi, within the body. From the perspective of modern science, acupuncture stimulates the release of endorphins, the body's natural painkillers, and affects the part of the brain that governs serotonin, a neurotransmitter implicated in mood and pain. Clinical trials have lent credence to the effectiveness of acupuncture in reducing fibromyalgia symptoms, marking it as a valuable component of a holistic treatment plan. The experience of acupuncture, for many, transcends the physical, offering moments of profound relaxation and a deepened connection to the body's innate capacity for healing.

Nutritional adjustments, while modest in their approach, wield a profound influence on the experience of fibromyalgia. The intricate relationship between diet and inflammation underpins this aspect of treatment, with certain foods known to exacerbate inflammatory processes and others capable of quitting them. Adopting an anti-inflammatory diet, rich in fruits, vegetables, whole grains, and lean proteins, aligns with this understanding, providing the body with the nutrients it needs to combat inflammation and potentially reduce the severity of fibromyalgia symptoms. This dietary strategy, supported by emerging research, offers individuals control over their symptomatology, empowering them through choices made at the dining table. The adjustments required extend beyond mere food selection, encompassing meal timing, portion sizes, and the integration of supplements to address nutritional deficiencies that may amplify fibromyalgia symptoms.

The philosophy of integrative medicine, which espouses a comprehensive approach to care by blending conventional and alternative therapies, underscores the potential of these nonpharmacological treatments. This model recognizes the multifaceted nature of fibromyalgia and the need for a treatment plan that addresses not just the physical symptoms but also the emotional and psychological aspects of the condition. In this framework, physical therapy, acupuncture, and nutritional adjustments are not standalone interventions but parts of a cohesive strategy that prioritizes the individual's overall wellbeing. The integrative approach fosters collaboration among healthcare providers, ensuring that each aspect of treatment is harmonized with the others, amplifying the potential for relief, and enhancing the quality of care.

Navigating the realm of nonpharmacological treatments necessitates guidance from practitioners experienced in the nuances of fibromyalgia management. Identifying these professionals begins with a dialogue with one's primary care physician, a conversation that opens the door to referrals and recommendations. Researching local and online fibromyalgia support groups also yields insights into practitioners who have garnered positive feedback from the fibromyalgia community. When evaluating potential providers, inquiries about their experience with fibromyalgia, their approach to treatment, and their philosophy regarding patient care are essential. While requiring time and discernment, this vetting process leads to forming a care team tuned to the individual's needs, experienced in managing fibromyalgia, and committed to an integrated approach to healing.

In this exploration of nonpharmacological treatments for fibromyalgia, the journey transcends the quest for symptom relief, venturing into the realm of holistic care. Physical therapy, acupuncture, and nutritional adjustments, grounded in evidence and woven into the fabric of integrative medicine, offer avenues for managing fibromyalgia that respect the complexity of the condition. This approach, characterized by collaboration, individualization, and a commitment to treating the whole person, embodies the ethos of fibromyalgia management—a journey not defined by the search for a cure but by the pursuit of wellbeing and the challenges of living with chronic pain.

7.5 Tackling Isolation: Building Your Fibromyalgia Support Network

The specter of isolation looms large in the lives of those contending with fibromyalgia, a silent adversary that amplifies the physical discomfort and emotional turmoil inherent to the condition. This isolation, born from a complex interplay between societal misconceptions, personal withdrawal, and the invisible nature of the ailment, often serves to exacerbate fibromyalgia symptoms, weaving a deeper layer of distress into the fabric of everyday existence. Acknowledging the critical role social support plays in mitigating this isolation becomes a vital step in crafting an integrated approach to managing fibromyalgia, one that transcends the physical to embrace the emotional and social dimensions of wellness.

In the quest to forge connections, fibromyalgia support groups emerge as sanctuaries of understanding and empathy, spaces where shared experiences serve as the foundation for deep, meaningful relationships. These groups in physical and digital realms offer a platform for exchanging stories, strategies, and solace, creating a collective wellspring of resilience. For those newly navigating the waters of fibromyalgia, these communities provide invaluable insights into the nuances of the condition, from navigating healthcare systems to identifying effective coping mechanisms. More importantly, they offer a mirror reflecting many experiences, a reminder that one is not alone in this struggle.

Online communities extend the reach of support, transcending geographical limitations to connect individuals across the globe. Platforms such as forums, social media groups, and blogs foster a sense of belonging, providing a lifeline for those who find physical attendance at support groups challenging due to the constraints of pain or mobility. These digital spaces, animated by the voices of countless individuals sharing their journeys, become a repository of collective wisdom, a source of comfort and guidance accessible from the confines of one's home.

Engaging with family and friends about the realities of fibromyalgia presents its own set of challenges and opportunities. Nuanced and ongoing communication serves as the bridge over the chasm of misunderstanding that often surrounds invisible illnesses. Initiating conversations that elucidate the multifaceted nature of fibromyalgia—its unpredictable flare-ups, the spectrum of symptoms, and the impact on daily life—invites those close to the individual to step into their world, fostering empathy and support. While sometimes challenging, these dialogues lay the groundwork for a supportive home environment, where accommodation is made not out of obligation but out of genuine care and understanding.

Moreover, educating loved ones on how they can offer support—be it through assistance with daily tasks, accompanying visits to healthcare providers, or simply providing a listening ear—empowers them to become active participants in managing fibromyalgia. This active participation not only alleviates the practical burdens of the condition but also reinforces the emotional bonds between the individual and their support network, weaving a more robust fabric of communal resilience.

Volunteer work and social activities stand as potent antidotes to the isolation fibromyalgia engenders, offering pathways to engagement and purpose that extend beyond the confines of the condition. Volunteering provides an avenue for individuals to transcend their own experiences, contributing to the welfare of others and, in the process, finding a sense of fulfillment and self-worth that fibromyalgia often obscures. Whether lending their time and skills to local charities, support groups, or community projects, individuals find these activities not only a distraction from pain but also a connection to a cause greater than themselves.

Social activities, tailored to accommodate the limitations fibromyalgia imposes, offer another venue for combating isolation. Participating in low-impact exercise classes, joining book clubs, or attending workshops on topics of interest fosters social interaction and provides an outlet for creativity and learning. These engagements, carefully selected to align with one's physical capabilities and interests, broaden the social circle, introducing individuals to peers who, while not sharing the experience of fibromyalgia, bring diversity of thought and companionship into their lives.

The construction of a fibromyalgia support network, multifaceted in its composition, emerges as a cornerstone of effective management, addressing the emotional and social dimensions of the condition. This network, built through deliberate steps to connect with others, navigate relationships, and engage in volunteer work and social activities, is a bulwark against isolation. It underscores the importance of community and connection in navigating the complexities of fibromyalgia, reinforcing the idea that while pain may be a constant companion, one need not face it alone. Through these connections, individuals forge a path marked not by solitude but by shared understanding and support, a journey made lighter by the presence of others.

7.6 Coping with Flare-Ups: Practical Tips and Emotional Support

An intrinsic part of navigating life with fibromyalgia involves the unpredictable onset of flare-ups, where symptoms intensify without warning, casting shadows over days that might otherwise feel manageable. Recognizing the precursors to these episodes and understanding their unique triggers becomes a critical skill, akin to reading the signs of an approaching storm. For many, a subtle shift in weather patterns, a slight deviation from routine activities, or an unexpected emotional stressor can herald the onset of a flare-up. One can maintain control even in uncharted waters by tuning these signals, acknowledging their potential impact, and adjusting one's sails accordingly.

Crafting an emergency plan for these inevitable occurrences entails a meticulous gathering of resources and strategies, a kit of sorts that one can reach for when the tumult begins. This plan might include a list of medications proven to alleviate symptoms, complete with dosage and timing instructions to ensure optimal efficacy. Alongside pharmaceutical aids, a repertoire of relaxation techniques stands ready to deploy, from guided imagery exercises that transport one to calmer shores to deep breathing routines that anchor the body amidst the storm. Essential is the assembly of a support circle, individuals who can be called upon when self-navigation through a flare-up feels beyond one's capacity. This circle might consist of healthcare providers, family members, or close friends, each briefed on how best to assist during these challenging times.

Emotional resilience, the ability to weather the internal storms accompanying flare-ups, rests on foundations built from self-compassion and the pursuit of comfort in small, soothing activities. Engaging in acts of kindness towards oneself, recognizing the legitimacy of the pain, and allowing space for rest and recovery without guilt cultivates an environment where healing can commence. Comforting activities, those small oases of pleasure—immersing in a favorite book, listening to cherished music, or savoring a cup of tea—are gentle reminders of the joys that persist even in pain's shadow. These practices do not negate the reality of the flare-up but offer a counterbalance, a means to hold onto one's sense of self amidst the upheaval.

Long-term management of flare-ups transcends the immediate strategies employed in their midst, delving into the realm of lifestyle and treatment adjustments based on observed patterns and triggers. This adaptive approach is the gradual incorporation of a gentle exercise regimen designed to strengthen the body without overtaxing its limits. Dietary adjustments also play a role, emphasizing anti-inflammatory foods that support the body's natural defenses against pain and fatigue. The meticulous tracking of activities, stressors, and their corresponding impact on one's symptoms can illuminate trends over time, guiding the refinement of treatment and coping strategies to mitigate the frequency and intensity of flare-ups. This process, iterative and personalized, fosters a deeper understanding of one's condition, empowering informed decisions about care and management.

In the face of fibromyalgia's unpredictability, the strategies outlined here offer not a panacea but a framework for resilience, a means to navigate flare-ups with grace and grit. Recognizing triggers and warning signs, crafting a personalized emergency plan, cultivating emotional resilience, and adjusting lifestyle and treatment strategies based on observed patterns constitute a comprehensive approach to managing flare-ups. These practices, woven into the fabric of daily life, provide a bulwark against the tempests of fibromyalgia, ensuring that even in the storm's grasp, one retains a measure of control and a connection to the enduring spirit that defines the human experience.

As we draw this chapter close, the emphasis on practicality and support in managing fibromyalgia flare-ups stands clear. The path laid out, from understanding triggers to crafting emergency plans, fostering emotional resilience, and adjusting lifestyle choices, offers a guide through the tumultuous periods of intensified symptoms. Though personal and unique in its challenges, this journey is underscored by the universal need for preparation, support, and self-compassion. Moving forward, the focus shifts towards a broader exploration of strategies and insights, each step aimed at enhancing the journey through fibromyalgia with knowledge, support, and hope.

Chapter 8 Real Women, Real Success: Stories of Overcoming Fibromyalgia

In the tapestry of fibromyalgia management, stories of triumph resonate with a unique power, illuminating the path for others still navigating the fog of chronic pain. These narratives, each distinct in their struggles and victories, serve as beacons of hope, demonstrating the profound impact of resilience, creativity, and community support in the face of fibromyalgia. They underscore a vital truth: while the condition may shape aspects of one's life, it does not define it in totality.

Diverse Experiences, Unified Hope

Across the globe, women from varied backgrounds confront fibromyalgia's challenges daily. Their stories, rich in detail and emotion, paint a vivid picture of the fight against chronic pain. Consider a teacher who, despite the constant ache in her bones, finds solace and strength in her students' smiles, using her breaks to practice mindfulness techniques that allow her to stay present and engaged. Or a grandmother who, facing the sharp stings of fibromyalgia, channels her energy into creating a garden, a visual metaphor for growth and resilience, finding a connection to life's renewal cycles in the soil. These stories, while highlighting the individuality of each experience, weave a common thread of hope, showing that life, though altered, continues richly and fully.

Textual Element: Reflection Section
- Reflect on a moment of triumph over your fibromyalgia symptoms. What strategies helped you through?
- Identify a daily activity that brings you joy and consider how it can be adapted to accommodate your condition.

Lessons Learned

The journey through fibromyalgia is punctuated with lessons and hard-earned insights that become guiding lights. Key among these is the understanding that self-care is not selfish but necessary, a foundation upon which wellness is built. This lesson, often realized through trial and error, emphasizes listening to one's body, recognizing its limits and signals, and responding with kindness. The practice of pacing, breaking tasks into manageable chunks, and interspersing rest periods emerges as a critical strategy, allowing for productivity without worsening symptoms. Additionally, the power of community, found in support groups and online forums, is revealed as an invaluable resource, providing practical advice, emotional solace, and understanding.

The Role of Perseverance

Perseverance, the quiet determination underpinning each story of success, proves essential in managing fibromyalgia. It is the force that propels one to seek new treatments, experiment with dietary changes, or adopt a new exercise regimen despite the uncertainty of outcomes. This perseverance is fueled by a belief in possibility, in the potential for better days, and is strengthened by each small victory, whether it is a pain-free afternoon or a restful night's sleep. It is a reminder that while fibromyalgia may present a formidable opponent, the human spirit, fortified by hope and tenacity, possesses remarkable resilience.

Inspiration for Action

The stories of women who have navigated the complexities of fibromyalgia and emerged with lives full of purpose and joy serve as a clarion call to action. They invite others still in the throes of pain to look beyond their current circumstances to envision a future where fibromyalgia is but one facet of a vibrant life. These narratives encourage the exploration of new hobbies that accommodate physical limitations, pursuing passions that had been sidelined, and forging connections with others who understand the journey. They demonstrate that managing fibromyalgia, while undoubtedly challenging, also offers opportunities for growth, self-discovery, and deepened relationships.

The essence of these success stories lies not in eradicating symptoms but in the ability to live fully despite them. They offer proof that with the right combination of treatments, lifestyle adjustments, and support, fibromyalgia can be managed, and life can be lived with richness and depth. These stories do not promise an easy path but offer the assurance that it is worth taking, filled with potential for fulfillment and joy.

In sharing these experiences, the aim is not only to educate and inform but to ignite a spark of hope and determination in those still searching for their path through fibromyalgia. It is an invitation to view each day not as a battle to be fought but as an opportunity to be embraced, with all its challenges and rewards. These stories stand as a testament to the power of resilience, creativity, and community in transforming the experience of living with fibromyalgia, offering a beacon of hope for all who journey with this condition.

8.1 Setting and Achieving Personal Wellness Goals

In the realm where fibromyalgia's shadows loom, setting and achieving personal wellness goals becomes a tapestry of intention and resilience. This tapestry, interwoven with the threads of aspirations and practical strategies, maps out a landscape where goals are envisioned and pursued with a purpose tailored to the contours of living with a chronic condition. The process, nuanced and deeply personal, balances ambition with the realities of fibromyalgia, crafting a pathway where progress, in any measure, is celebrated.

Goal-setting Principles

The architecture of effective goal setting in the context of fibromyalgia management is built upon principles that honor the individual's current state while reaching toward an envisioned future. At its core, this architecture respects the variability of the condition, acknowledging that a symphony of pain and fatigue marks some days while others hum with a quieter intensity. Goals, therefore, are mapped with flexibility, allowing for the ebb and flow of symptoms, and are rooted in a deep understanding of one's capacities and limits. This understanding informs the selection of goals that are not only desirable but attainable, framing aspirations within the realm of the possible.

SMART Goals for Health

The SMART framework, a beacon in the goal-setting process, illuminates the path toward wellness, emphasizing specificity, measurability, achievability, relevance, and time-bound criteria. In the landscape of fibromyalgia management, this framework takes on a nuanced significance, guiding the individual in sculpting goals that are finely tuned to the rhythms of their condition. A goal could be as specific as integrating a ten-minute meditation practice into the morning routine, measured by its duration and consistency and impact on the day's pain levels. Achievability is gauged against current capabilities, ensuring that goals stretch the individual's limits without straining them. Relevance emerges through aligning goals with personal values and wellness aspirations, ensuring that each step forward resonates with the individual's broader vision for life. Time-bound criteria introduce a dimension of urgency and structure, setting a framework within which progress can be assessed and celebrated.

Celebrating Milestones
In the journey toward wellness, milestones serve as lanterns along the path, casting light on progress and illuminating the way forward. These milestones, whether they mark the consistent practice of a new skill, the successful management of a particularly challenging flare-up, or the integration of a dietary change, are moments of triumph over the adversities of fibromyalgia. Celebrating these milestones fosters a sense of achievement and bolsters the spirit, fueling the motivation to continue. In this context, celebration transcends the act of acknowledgment, becoming a ritual of appreciation for the resilience and effort that each milestone represents.

Adjusting Goals as Needed
The landscape of fibromyalgia is marked by its unpredictability, a terrain where symptoms shift like the weather, and what was achievable one day may become a mountain the next. This variability necessitates flexibility in goal setting, achievement, and openness to adjust aspirations as the condition ebbs and flows. Adjustments may mean scaling back on the intensity of physical activities, extending timelines for specific objectives, or redefining success in the context of new limitations. This process, far from signaling defeat, reflects a responsive and compassionate approach to self-care that honors the body's signals and adapts to its needs. It underscores the dynamic nature of living with fibromyalgia, where goals are not static landmarks but guideposts along a winding path, subject to change as the journey unfolds.

In setting and achieving personal wellness goals amidst the complexities of fibromyalgia, individuals craft a narrative of resilience and hope. This narrative, punctuated by practical goal-setting principles, the SMART framework's strategic application, the celebration of milestones, and the flexibility to adjust goals as needed, charts a course toward enhanced wellbeing. It is a course that acknowledges the challenges of the condition while affirming the individual's capacity to shape their journey, a testament to the power of intention, strategy, and perseverance in the quest for a fulfilling life with fibromyalgia.

8.2 The Role of Continuous Learning in Fibromyalgia Management

Staying informed stands as a beacon for those navigating the murky waters of fibromyalgia, illuminating a path through the dense fog of uncertainty that envelops the condition. This illumination is not merely about casting light on the shadows of the unknown but about fostering a landscape where empowerment and self-advocacy take root and flourish. The realm of fibromyalgia, with its ever-shifting contours and hidden depths, demands a vigilant eye and a curious mind, ready to absorb the latest research, treatments, and strategies from the scientific community. This pursuit of knowledge, however, extends beyond the confines of personal gain; it is a shared journey where every piece of information, every discovery, holds the potential to light the way for others lost in the dark. Leveraging resources becomes an act of navigation, a skill honed through the discerning selection of reputable sources of information. Medical journals, peer-reviewed and steeped in rigorous research, offer a wellspring of knowledge, presenting findings from the latest studies in a language that bridges the gap between the complexities of science and the thirst for understanding. Patient advocacy groups and educational websites, curated by those who have traversed the path of fibromyalgia themselves, provide a compass by which to steer, offering guidance, support, and a sense of community. These carefully chosen and critically examined resources serve as the building blocks for a foundation of knowledge upon which decisions about treatment and management can be confidently made.

Learning from others, an exercise in humility and openness acknowledges that wisdom often resides in the lived experiences of those who walk the path alongside us. The exchange of stories, tips, and encouragement in forums, support groups, and informal gatherings becomes a tapestry of collective knowledge, rich in the nuances of personal triumphs and setbacks. Each shared experience, each piece of advice passed from one to another, is a thread in this tapestry, adding strength and color to the collective understanding of fibromyalgia. This process of communal learning, an organic flow of give-and-take, not only broadens the individual's perspective but also reinforces the bonds that connect those affected by the condition, creating a network of support that spans the globe.

Empowerment through education emerges as the cornerstone of this collective journey, a principle that elevates the quest for knowledge from a passive activity to an active pursuit of agency. Armed with information, individuals find themselves better equipped to engage in dialogues with healthcare providers, question, challenge, and collaborate in creating treatment plans that reflect their unique needs and experiences. This empowerment, however, transcends the clinical setting, extending its reach into the daily lives of those with fibromyalgia. It manifests in the choices made at the grocery store, the selection of physical activities, and the crafting of routines that align with the body's rhythms and limitations. It is a force that transforms victims into advocates, passive recipients of care, and active participants in the journey toward wellness.

In this landscape of continuous learning, the horizon is ever-expanding, offering vistas of hope and possibility to those willing to seek them out. The commitment to staying informed, leveraging resources, learning from others, and finding empowerment through education is not a solitary endeavor but a collective voyage. It is a testament to the resilience of the human spirit, a reaffirmation of the belief that growth, understanding, and empowerment are within reach even in the face of chronic pain and uncertainty.

8.3 Embracing a New Normal: Life Beyond Fibromyalgia Pain

In the quiet aftermath of a fibromyalgia diagnosis, the landscape of one's identity often undergoes a subtle yet profound transformation. No longer merely individuals navigating the complexities of life, people find themselves adorned with a new descriptor – that of a fibromyalgia patient. While offering a semblance of understanding and community, this label can also cast a shadow over the vibrant mosaic of traits, achievements, and dreams that comprise one's true self. The challenge lies not in accepting this new aspect of existence but in the refusal to let it eclipse the totality of one's identity.

Redefining oneself after such a diagnosis involves a deliberate act of will, a conscious decision to focus on the strengths, interests, and passions that persist despite the condition's presence. This redefinition is akin to the careful cultivation of a garden, where the weeds of doubt and limitation are diligently removed to allow the flourishing of one's inherent qualities and aspirations. It is a process of introspection, of peeling away the layers of fibromyalgia to reveal the core of who one truly is – an individual not defined by pain but characterized by the resilience, creativity, and determination that pain has failed to extinguish.

The adaptation to life changes brought about by fibromyalgia mirrors the acclimatization process to a new climate, where initial discomfort gives way to a newfound appreciation for the nuances of this altered state of being. Activities once taken for granted may now require modification, a recalibration of expectations, and methods to align with the body's fluctuating capabilities. Yet, within this adaptation lies the opportunity for innovation and discovery, for finding new avenues of joy and fulfillment that resonate with one's current reality. It is a journey of experimentation, where the exploration of alternative hobbies, the modification of favorite pastimes, and the adoption of new routines become acts of defiance against the restrictions imposed by fibromyalgia.

Maintaining a positive outlook in such a pervasive condition is akin to navigating by the stars in a storm-tossed sea. The practice of gratitude, a deliberate focus on the elements of life that remain untarnished by pain, serves as a compass in this endeavor. This practice may manifest in the simple acknowledgment of a pain-free moment, the warmth of sunlight on one's face, or the support of a loved one – each a beacon of hope in the darker moments. Moreover, the concentration on aspects of life within one's control, from the management of symptoms through lifestyle choices to the engagement in meaningful activities, imbues individuals with a sense of agency, a reminder that, despite the unpredictability of fibromyalgia, they remain captains of their ships.

Planning for the future amidst the uncertainties of fibromyalgia requires a balance of optimism and realism, a navigation between the shores of hope and the rocky outcrops of practicality. Setting long-term goals in this context becomes an act of defiance, a declaration of belief in one's ability to shape the future despite the condition's attempts to dictate the course. These goals, be they related to personal achievements, relationships, or professional endeavors, are charged with an awareness of potential obstacles yet are pursued with a determination that acknowledges no barrier as insurmountable. The planning process, flexible and adaptive, allows for the shifting sands of fibromyalgia, accommodating fluctuations in health while steadfastly progressing toward the envisioned horizon.

In embracing this new normal, individuals forge a path through the wilderness of fibromyalgia, marked by the redefinition of identity, the adaptation to life changes, the maintenance of a positive outlook, and the forward gaze toward future aspirations. Though fraught with challenges, this path is also lined with opportunities for growth, self-discovery, and the deepening of connections with others. It is a testament to the indomitable spirit of those who, faced with the disruption of chronic pain, choose not merely to endure but to thrive, crafting lives of richness and depth in the shadow of fibromyalgia.

8.4 Expanding Your Toolkit: When to Seek Additional Help

In the vast and often turbulent sea of fibromyalgia management, there comes a time when the sails of self-guided strategies no longer catch the wind as they once did. During these moments, when familiar shoes fade into the mist, the call for additional assistance echoes most loudly. Recognizing this need for reinforcement or adjustment in one's approach is not a sign of failure but rather an acknowledgment of the condition's complexity. The initial step in this process involves a candid self-assessment and a quiet but profound conversation with oneself about the effectiveness of current management strategies. This inner dialogue probes the depths of one's resilience, questioning whether the pain, fatigue and other accompanying symptoms have begun to breach the bulwarks of daily routines and emotional wellbeing. Now, it is here that the contemplation of expanding one's toolkit begins, opening the door to previously untraveled avenues.

The realm of therapy and counseling offers a sanctuary for those seeking solace from the psychological burdens that fibromyalgia invariably brings. The benefits of engaging with mental health professionals extend beyond the confines of traditional therapy; they provide a space where the tangled threads of anxiety, depression, and stress, often interwoven with the physical pain of fibromyalgia, can be gently unraveled. Therapists specializing in chronic pain management possess the unique ability to navigate these intricate emotional landscapes, guiding their clients toward strategies that foster resilience, acceptance, and a sense of peace. Moreover, the exploration of cognitive-behavioral therapy offers a structured approach to reshaping the thought patterns that may exacerbate one's experience of pain, transforming the mind into an ally rather than an adversary in the management of fibromyalgia.

As one ventures further into the expanse of potential treatments, the allure of alternative therapies becomes increasingly palpable. Biofeedback, a technique that trains individuals to control physiological processes such as heart rate and muscle tension, emerges as a beacon for those seeking to reclaim autonomy over their bodies. Through the subtle art of awareness and modulation, biofeedback empowers individuals to temper their physiological responses to stress and pain, offering a semblance of relief in the face of fibromyalgia's unpredictability. Similarly, massage therapy, with its ancient roots and myriad forms, provides not only a reprieve from muscle stiffness and soreness but also a momentary escape from the relentless grip of chronic pain. These therapies, while diverse in their methodologies, share a common goal: to alleviate the physical and emotional burdens of fibromyalgia, offering a glimpse of tranquility amidst the storm.

Navigating the multifaceted landscape of healthcare services for specialist support presents challenges and opportunities. The quest for a rheumatologist or pain management clinic well-versed in the subtleties of fibromyalgia requires diligence, patience, and, often, a willingness to advocate fiercely for one's health. This voyage begins with gathering recommendations from primary care providers, fellow fibromyalgia patients, or reputable medical associations. Armed with this information, individuals embark on a series of consultations, each an opportunity to assess the compatibility of the specialist's approach with their own needs and values. Questions concerning the specialist's experience with fibromyalgia, their philosophy regarding patient involvement in treatment decisions, and their openness to integrating alternative therapies alongside conventional treatments become compass points guiding the decision-making process. Through this meticulous exploration of healthcare services, individuals forge partnerships with providers, crafting a collaborative and integrated approach to fibromyalgia management.

In the endeavor to expand one's toolkit for managing fibromyalgia, the journey from recognizing the need for additional help to engaging with the breadth of available resources is marked by introspection, exploration, and a steadfast commitment to self-advocacy. This process, though daunting in its scope, is illuminated by the promise of discovering new strategies that resonate with one's unique circumstances, offering a renewed sense of hope and control. As individuals traverse this landscape, guided by an unwavering determination to seek relief, and enhance their quality of life, the horizon of fibromyalgia management broadens, revealing a vista of possibilities previously obscured by the shadows of pain and uncertainty.

8.5 Celebrating Every Victory: Big or Small

Amidst the fluctuating tides of fibromyalgia, recognizing and celebrating every triumph, no matter its magnitude, emerges as a beacon of light. This light illuminates the path traversed and scatters the shadows of doubt and Despair that often accompany chronic conditions. The acknowledgment of achievements, from the minutiae of daily victories to the significant milestones of progress, serves as a testament to the resilience and fortitude that define the human spirit when faced with adversity. Within this acknowledgment, a profound sense of empowerment is nurtured, fostering a mindset attuned to the possibilities of growth and the potential for joy that exists in each moment.

Encouraging the sharing of successes with one's support network casts ripples across the waters of isolation, creating waves of inspiration and encouragement that touch the lives of others navigating similar journeys. This simple yet profound gesture of sharing becomes a conduit for connection, a bridge spanning the distances between individuals, allowing them to draw strength from shared experiences. It transforms personal victories into communal triumphs, weaving a tapestry of collective resilience that blankets the community with hope. As these stories of success are shared, they become beacons for others, guiding them through their darkest hours and reminding them of the light that persists amidst the pain.

The suggestion to maintain a victory journal introduces a tangible element to the practice of acknowledgment, providing a sanctuary for thoughts and reflections. Within its pages, the chronicles of achievements, breakthroughs, and moments of joy are preserved, serving as a mirror reflecting the journey's highs and lows. This journal, a mosaic of grand and humble triumphs, becomes a source of motivation and reflection, a tool for navigating the emotional landscapes of fibromyalgia. It allows for tracking progress over time, offering concrete evidence of the strides made, and serves as a reminder of the capacity for growth and adaptation that dwells within.

Discussing the cumulative effect of small wins unveils the profound impact these victories have on the overall quality of life and wellbeing. Each success, no matter its scale, contributes to a foundation of confidence and optimism, gradually altering the perception of one's capabilities and the nature of the condition itself. When woven together, these incremental achievements form a fabric of resilience that drapes over the challenges of fibromyalgia, softening their impact and imbuing the individual with a sense of accomplishment and purpose. Through this accumulation of victories, a transformation occurs, not in the condition itself but in how it is perceived and confronted. The aggregate of these triumphs fosters a climate of positivity and hope, proving that even in the face of chronic pain, there exists a wellspring of potential for fulfillment and happiness.

This chapter, a mosaic of strategies and reflections, weaves together the threads of acknowledgment, sharing, journaling, and the recognition of incremental progress into a tapestry that celebrates the human ability for resilience. It underscores the importance of embracing every victory and understanding that each success, whether whispered or declared, contributes to the broader narrative of managing fibromyalgia. In doing so, it invites readers to view their journey not as a series of obstacles but as an opportunity for growth, connection, and self-discovery.

Conclusion

Embarking on the journey through these pages, we have traversed the terrain of fibromyalgia together, uncovering the profound effectiveness of Cognitive Behavioral Therapy (CBT) and meditation in managing the pain that so often clouds our days. We delved deep into the holistic approach, illuminating how the synergy of diet modifications, gentle exercise, and a steadfast positive mindset forms the cornerstone of a comprehensive strategy aimed at alleviating symptoms and enhancing quality of life.

As we stand now, it is vital to reflect on this journey not merely as a quest for symptom management but as a profound opportunity for discovery and empowerment. Each chapter was crafted to equip you with the tools for advocacy and continuous learning to navigate the complexities of fibromyalgia with confidence and grace.

From understanding the multifaceted impact of fibromyalgia and the transformative power of CBT and meditation to the practical guides for incorporating diet and physical activity into your daily regimen, the key takeaways from each section are steppingstones on your path to resilience. These strategies, illuminated with real stories of triumph and perseverance, serve as beacons of hope, reinforcing that while the path may be fraught with challenges, the strength resides within you.

Our collective narrative emphasizes the significance of personalizing your management plan. There is a unique blend of strategies that will resonate with your circumstances, and I encourage you to approach this with an open heart and mind. Begin your journey towards better-managing fibromyalgia today, armed with the insights and strategies shared within these pages. Embrace patience, celebrate every small victory, and remember that progress is a monumental step forward, no matter how incremental.

I acknowledge the road ahead may have its share of hurdles but let us keep sight of the potential for remarkable improvements in managing pain and enhancing our quality of life.

Your dedication, coupled with the right strategies, can pave the way for a future where fibromyalgia no longer dictates the terms of your existence.

Thank you for allowing me to be a part of your journey. Remember, you are not navigating this path alone. The fibromyalgia community, healthcare professionals, and resources mentioned throughout this book are your allies, ready to offer support and guidance.

As we bring this chapter to a close, I urge you to continue exploring, learning, and adapting. Stay abreast of the latest research, remain active in your healthcare decisions, and never hesitate to seek new avenues for managing your symptoms. Managing fibromyalgia is an evolving process, one that, with perseverance and optimism, can lead to a life defined not by pain but by the joy and fulfillment found in overcoming it.

Together, let us step forward with hope, resilience, and a relentless spirit of discovery. The journey to managing fibromyalgia is paved with challenges. Still, it is also ripe with the potential for growth, empowerment, and a deeper appreciation for the strength within us all.

The seven steps to reduce Fibromyalgia pain through CBT Therapy are

Step One- Diet and Hydration for fibromyalgia health (chapter 2)

Step Two- Pain Management Plan for fibromyalgia (chapter 2)

Step Three- Support System (chapters 3 and 8)

Step Four- Meditation and Deep Breathing (chapter 4 and 5)

Step Five- Getting Proper Rest (chapter 6)

Step Six- Easy Exercise for Fibromyalgia (chapter 6)

Step Seven- Incremental change and Goal setting (chapters 7 & 8).

Good Luck On your Journey to manage Fibromyalgia!

References
- *Gender Differences in the Prevalence of Fibromyalgia and ...*
  https://www.ncbi.nlm.nih.gov/pmc/articles/PMC6425926/
- *Why Women Are More Prone to Fibromyalgia: Dr. Lenny Cohen*
  https://www.chicagoneurodoc.com/blog/why-women-are-more-prone-to-fibromyalgia#:~:text=Estrogen%20may%20influence%20your%20pain,your%20pain%20sensitivity%20may%20increase.
- *Facts and myths about fibromyalgia - PMC*
  https://www.ncbi.nlm.nih.gov/pmc/articles/PMC6016048/
- *Coping with fibromyalgia - a focus group study - PMC*
  https://www.ncbi.nlm.nih.gov/pmc/articles/PMC10120560/

- *Nutritional Interventions in the Management of Fibromyalgia*
  https://www.ncbi.nlm.nih.gov/pmc/articles/PMC7551285/
- *Cognitive-behavioral therapy for patients with chronic pain*
  https://www.ncbi.nlm.nih.gov/pmc/articles/PMC5999451/
- *Mindfulness Meditation for Fibromyalgia: Mechanistic and ...*
  https://www.ncbi.nlm.nih.gov/pmc/articles/PMC5693231/
- *Combining Mindfulness Meditation with Cognitive ...*
  https://www.ncbi.nlm.nih.gov/pmc/articles/PMC3052789/
- *Cognitive-behavioral therapy for patients with chronic pain*
  https://www.ncbi.nlm.nih.gov/pmc/articles/PMC5999451/
- *Cognitive Biases in Chronic Illness and Their Impact on ...*
  https://www.ncbi.nlm.nih.gov/pmc/articles/PMC7655771/
- *Goals of Chronic Pain Management: Do Patients and ...*
  https://www.ncbi.nlm.nih.gov/pmc/articles/PMC5572549/
- *Using cognitive behavior therapy to explore resilience in ...*
  https://www.ncbi.nlm.nih.gov/pmc/articles/PMC5047334/
- *Mindfulness meditation-based pain relief: a mechanistic ...*
  https://www.ncbi.nlm.nih.gov/pmc/articles/PMC4941786/
- *Mindfulness Meditation for Fibromyalgia: Mechanistic and ...*
  https://www.ncbi.nlm.nih.gov/pmc/articles/PMC5693231/
- *Effect of guided imagery on anxiety, muscle pain, and vital ...*
  https://www.ncbi.nlm.nih.gov/pmc/articles/PMC7982304/
- *Effects of progressive muscle relaxation therapy at home ...*
  https://pubmed.ncbi.nlm.nih.gov/34151818/
- *Neuroscience Reveals the Secrets of Meditation's Benefits*
  https://www.scientificamerican.com/article/neuroscience-reveals-the-secrets-of-meditation-s-benefits/
- *Using Yoga Nidra to manage pain - practice*
  https://www.ekhartyoga.com/videos/using-yoga-nidra-to-manage-pain-practice
- *Loving-Kindness Meditation to Target Affect in Mood ...*
  https://www.ncbi.nlm.nih.gov/pmc/articles/PMC4468348/
- *How to Practice Zazen* https://www.lionsroar.com/how-to-practice-zazen/
- *Fibromyalgia and Sleep: Sleep Disturbances & Coping*
  https://www.sleepfoundation.org/physical-health/fibromyalgia-and-sleep
- *Fibromyalgia Pain Relief with Stretching and Strength Exercises*
  https://www.webmd.com/fibromyalgia/ss/slideshow-fibromyalgia-friendly-exercises

- *Fibromyalgia Diet: Eating to Ease Symptoms - Healthline*
  https://www.healthline.com/health/fibromyalgia-diet-to-ease-symptoms
- *Fibromyalgia: Exercise, relaxation, and stress management*
  https://www.ncbi.nlm.nih.gov/books/NBK492990/
- *Can cognitive-behavioral therapy lessen fibromyalgia pain?*
  https://newsroom.wiley.com/press-releases/press-release-details/2023/Can-cognitive-behavioral-therapy-lessen-fibromyalgia-pain/default.aspx
- *Mindfulness meditation-based pain relief: a mechanistic ...*
  https://www.ncbi.nlm.nih.gov/pmc/articles/PMC4941786/
- *Efficacy of nonpharmacological interventions for individual...*
  https://journals.lww.com/pain/fulltext/2022/08000/efficacy_of_nonpharmacological_interventions_for.2.aspx
- *Building Peer Support Programs to Manage Chronic Disease*
  https://www.chcf.org/wp-content/uploads/2017/12/PDF-BuildingPeerSupportPrograms.pdf
- *Cindy Tedrow: Functional Medicine Patient Story*
  https://my.clevelandclinic.org/patient-stories/196-functional-medicine-helps-woman-regain-her-life-after-44-years-of-chronic-pain
- *Goal Setting for Pain Rehabilitation - Whole Health Library*
  https://www.va.gov/WHOLEHEALTHLIBRARY/tools/goal-setting-for-pain-rehabilitation.asp
- *2023's Breakthrough Fibromyalgia Treatments & Advances*
  https://www.dvcstem.com/post/new-treatments-for-fibromyalgia
- *Internet-Based Cognitive Behavioral Therapy for ...*
  https://www.ncbi.nlm.nih.gov/pmc/articles/PMC10197913/

Made in United States
Troutdale, OR
04/26/2025